Praise for *The Bathroom Key*

"Arnold Henry Kegel, MD, FACS, was my father and he made a substantial contribution in the field of medicine during his lifetime. Kegel exercises bear his name. His original work immeasurably improved the lives of women suffering from incontinence. The advanced techniques presented in this book work even better today—to eliminate incontinence once and for all…"
—Robert Arnold Kegel, Esq.

"This is a book for every mother, daughter and girlfriend. Kim and Kathryn describe not only their journey, but the journey of many real women. The information is understandable, and more importantly, applicable to every woman at every stage of their lives."
—Sarah Haag, PT, DPT, MS, WCS, Chicago, IL

"Authors Kassai and Perelli instill confidence that control over the bladder is achievable and resides within each of us. Hooray to both authors for putting into context the essential role played by physical therapy. They have assembled a no-nonsense, unbeatable set of guidelines and instructions for achieving not only continence but reclaiming one's entire pelvic health."
—Nancy Muller, PhD, Executive Director, National Association for Continence

"It is an amazing truth that most incontinent woman can become dry without surgery and without medicines. Pelvic floor muscle therapy and biofeedback, as described in this book, has become a powerfully effective standard tool in the fight against bladder dysfunction. As a Urologist, I love it when my incontinent patients become dry; when they can sleep through the night without getting up to urinate; when they don't have to know where every bathroom in the mall is before they can go shopping. This fabulous book reveals the physical therapy methods that can give people—with all sorts of bladder problems—their lives back. Read this book and it might just change your life."
—Fredrick N. Wolk, MD, Diplomat of the American Board of Urology

"*The Bathroom Key* is a wonderful resource for any woman with symptoms of urinary incontinence, pelvic prolapse, or issues of pelvic pain and discomfort with sexual activity. Kathryn and Kim do a great job describing why women may have these symptoms and discussing the various treatment options. I love the way they use real patients as examples throughout the book and explain everything in plain language without confusing the reader with medical terms which that can be hard to understand."
>   —**David A. Ginsberg, MD,** Associate Professor of Clinical Urology, USC Institute of Urology, Keck School of Medicine

"*The Bathroom Key* is a must-read for anyone over 20. It takes an embarrassing problem and turns it in to a controllable situation."
>   —**Pamela J. Rizzo,** Publisher, *The Women's Journal*

"I have been in Gynecological practice for 24 years and I have never seen a "compendium" on urinary incontinence for patients and physicians alike. What a service for millions of our patients who can use this information and seek treatment without embarrassment and shame. Thanks to Kathryn and Kim, incontinence is no longer a 'closet' medical issue. I plan to recommend this book to my patients."
>   —**Cecelia M. Hann, MD,** Gynecologist, Santa Clarita, CA

"This book is a fantastic resource with great information and real techniques for patients and professionals alike."
>   —**Isa Herrera, MSPT, CSCS,** Author of *Ending Female Pain: A Woman's Manual* and Owner of Renew Physical Therapy Healing Center, New York City

"*The Bathroom Key* is an essential book that all sufferers of urinary and/or fecal incontinence should own. It offers easy-to-follow exercises to reduce or eliminate pelvic floor weakness and pelvic floor dysfunction. Musculoskeletal causes of pelvic floor dysfunction are commonly misdiagnosed, and this book will give you clarification and lead you toward a proper diagnosis and treatment. I highly recommend this book and believe that it should be on the bookshelves of all OB/GYN and urological physicians!"
>   —**Amy Stein, MPT, BCB-PMD,** Board Member of the International Pelvic Pain Society, Author of *Heal Pelvic Pain*, Owner of Beyond Basics Physical Therapy, New York City

"Specific and readable—this timely pelvic health book is prime for the masses! Kathryn and Kim capture, with passion, the essence of why we do what we do as women's health physical therapists."
>—Jennifer Klestinski, PT, MPT, OCS, WCS, CSCS, BCB-PMD, Owner of CoreActive Therapy, LLC, Madison, WI

The Bathroom Key is a complete review of female pelvic health. Topics span incontinence, pelvic pain, and the mind-body connections. You'll get samples of exercise programs, practical behavioral tips, and techniques to eliminate symptoms. A great read to start you on your recovery journey."
>—Kathe Wallace, PT, BCB-PMD, International speaker, Consultant, Trainer, and Instructor in all aspects of physical therapy pelvic floor rehabilitation; Private Practice, Seattle, WA; Co-Founder of Herman and Wallace Pelvic Rehabilitation Institute

"This is a must-read book if you are a woman experiencing incontinence, frequent urinary tract infections, chronic pelvic pain, or pelvic organ prolapse. In clear, user-friendly language, with humor and inspiration, the authors give you the information and resources you need to vastly improve the quality of your life—a transformation I have seen occur in my patients treated by Kathryn. I urge you to read *The Bathroom Key*."
>—Joel Holtz, MD, Family Physician, Rancho Palos Verdes, CA

"At last, a book that explains the shifting paradigm in the understanding of overactive bladder and incontinence and—just as Kathryn and Kim do with their patients—gives the power of urinary control back to the patient. A well-structured and thoughtful work, *The Bathroom Key* unlocks the secrets to putting YOU in charge of your bladder, instead of vice versa. If you suffer from overactive bladder, urgency, prolapse, or any form of incontinence, this is a must-read."
>—Timothy Lesser, MD, Urologist, Torrance, CA

"I rarely find a physical therapy book that holds my attention from the very first page and that motivates me to read cover to cover in a week. This book did it for me! It is like reading an exciting novel that you can't wait to turn the page to find out what is going to happen next. It also takes you through an emotional journey by providing insights on what truly happens to our patients, in their attempts to create a semblance of normalcy despite their dysfunctions.

Tackling a subject that is considered 'taboo' across cultures, the collaborative writing of this book between a PT and a patient produced a product that is easy to read and that caters to patients, physicians, physical therapists, physical therapist assistants, and students. The authors transcended the concept of patient education to a new level in structuring the contents of the book and in their writing style. I wish that more therapists will take a cue from the authors and collaborate with their patients in writing textbooks to make them relatable and to 'humanize' the contents of their texts.

This book is truly a 'gift,' both to our profession and to our patients!"
—**Nelson Marquez, PT, EdD,** Physical Therapy Editor, *Today in PT Magazine,* Director, Physical Therapist Assistant Program, Polk State College

THE BATHROOM KEY

Put an End to Incontinence

Kathryn Kassai, Physical Therapist
and
Kim Perelli

Foreword by Jill G. Byers, MD

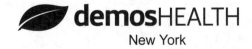 **demos**HEALTH

New York

Visit our website at www.demoshealth.com

ISBN:	978-1-936303-21-2
ebook ISBN:	978-1-617050-85-5

Acquisitions Editor: Noreen Henson
Compositor: Manila Typesetting Company

Medical information provided by Demos Health, in the absence of a visit with a healthcare professional, must be considered as an educational service only. This book is not designed to replace a physician's independent judgment about the appropriateness or risks of a procedure of therapy for a given patient. Our purpose is to provide you with information that will help you make your own healthcare decisions.

The information and opinions provided here are believed to be accurate and sound, based on the best judgment available to the authors, editors, and publisher, but readers who fail to consult appropriate health authorities assume the risk of injuries. The publisher is not responsible for errors or omissions. The editors and publisher welcome any reader to report to the publisher any discrepancies or inaccuracies noticed.

Library of Congress Cataloging-in-Publication Data
Kassai, Kathryn.
  The bathroom key : put an end to incontinence / Kathryn Kassai and Kim Perelli; foreword by Jill G. Byers.
      p. cm.
  Includes bibliographical references and index.
  ISBN 978-1-936303-21-2 (pbk.)
  1.   Urinary incontinence—Popular works. 2.   Urinary incontinence—Treatment—Popular works. I.   Perelli, Kim. II. Title.
  RC921.I5K37 2012
  616.6'2—dc23

                                                                    2011039060

Special discounts on bulk quantities of Demos Health books are available to corporations, professional associations, pharmaceutical companies, health care organizations, and other qualifying groups. For details, please contact:

Special Sales Department
Demos Medical Publishing
11 West 42nd Street, 15th Floor
New York, NY 10036
Phone: 800-532-8663 or 212-683-0072
Fax: 212-941-7842
E-mail: rsantana@demosmedpub.com

Printed in the United States of America by Bang Printing.
11 12 13 14 / 5 4 3 2 1

We dedicate THE BATHROOM KEY *to you, our readers. We understand how much courage it takes to venture out and seek resolution of your bladder woes.*

Contents

Acknowledging the Connection Between Incontinence and Depression
Becoming Whole Again
Your Home Program to Regain the Joy in Your Life

Foreword

As a physician, a surgeon, and one of the relatively few women in the field of Urology, I have found that the best thing about getting older is enjoying a broader perspective. The evolution of urinary incontinence treatment since my medical education began 25 years ago has been simply fascinating. I have become quite experienced in the management not only of urinary incontinence, but also pelvic prolapse, and pelvic pain.

Despite my extensive medical and surgical training in incontinence and other pelvic floor disorders, until I began developing my own experience in private practice, I had limited understanding of the role of physical therapy in treating those conditions. In contrast, I had learned dozens of different surgical procedures over this time, many of which have gone by the wayside, having been replaced by newer, improved versions. During this same period, implementation of physical therapy has continued to gain popularity, as study after study verifies its effectiveness.

The book you are holding in your hands represents the finest, most comprehensive work I have seen in the past 20 years. This book is not only welcome but overdue and, in my opinion, seminal (medical lingo for "earth shattering").

Whether you are suffering from urinary leakage (incontinence), frequent urination, vaginal prolapse, pelvic pain, or a combination of these, the tools described in exquisite detail, within this book, are tremendously valuable. After knowing Kathryn for 14 years, I remain stunned at the generosity of this veritable treasure trove on the pelvic floor. I also believe this book will prove to be extremely effective not only to the lay public, but also to practicing physicians, nurses, and physical therapists. Its comprehensiveness and readability will surely make it a classic.

To me, the best thing about being an experienced physician is witnessing firsthand how improved therapies come along and change patients' lives. I remain excited about my chosen field of Urology, because we have always been the under-recognized champions of less invasive, multifactorial treatment approaches. At the start of my medical practice, the term "biofeedback" was met with "bioWHAT?" and sounded like it was just "out there". But the principles of Dr. Arnold Kegel were built upon quietly and consistently, boosted by improved technology, and eventually created a very effective treatment option. As more and more "peer-reviewed" articles supported its effectiveness, insurance coverage hesitatingly followed, and biofeedback has now become well accepted.

Unfortunately, what we as physicians still do not have a good grasp of is the role of exercise, muscle training, therapeutic massage, and manipulation of the pelvic floor. Kathryn and Kim are quite correct that in medical school, even in a program with a heavy emphasis on Women's Health, physicians have typically received little to no education regarding the use of physical therapy to treat pelvic floor conditions.

However, like all physicians, we urologists are always striving to get MORE results for LESS—fewer side effects, less pain, and (especially in today's economy) less expense. Physical therapy makes so much sense on each of these fronts. Although we are not the first or only physicians to utilize physical therapy—and our awakening to its benefits is occurring gradually—I am confident this book will assist us in healing our patients, and I am immensely grateful to Kathryn and Kim for writing it.

Kathryn and Kim are truly on a quest to help the millions of women suffering from these conditions. For example, they have included special sections on *Pelvic Pain* and *Depression* (which often accompanies both incontinence and pelvic pain). They even point out the fascinating link between serotonin, depression, and incontinence. To say that I am impressed with the thoroughness of their research would be an understatement.

Although this is a book geared toward women, I have many male patients who have also benefited from the physical therapy approach described in this book. I remember, years ago, remarking that I had "discovered" that men also have bladders. For decades we urologists had directed treatment of male urinary symptoms solely at the prostate, overlooking the possibility that an overactive bladder could also be a culprit. More recently, I have realized that men also have pelvic floor muscles. In parallel fashion, I have begun to incorporate pelvic floor physical therapy into the treatment of male pelvic pain with remarkable results.

In contrast to the widely held stereotype of surgeons, I am very happy that Kim was cured without surgery, and I am pleased to have played my part in the creation of this book by referring Kim to Kathryn. Enjoy!

Jill G. Byers, MD
Board-Certified Urologist
Director, Southern California Continence Center
Newport Beach, California

Acknowledgments

Many times a day I realize how much my own life is built on the labours of my fellowmen, and how earnestly I must exert myself in order to give in return as much as I have received.

—Albert Einstein

We would be negligent not to start our thanks with the obvious: the women and men who bravely walk into Kathryn's clinic in the hope of finding help. They, collectively and individually, encouraged the creation of this book. We are indebted to the hundreds of referring physicians, who reassure their patients that physical therapy for incontinence does work. In particular, we must recognize Jill Byers, MD, who took that essential step of referring Kim to Kathryn, and then wrote such a compelling foreword to our book.

Next, we applaud the incomparable Jim Woods, Esq., who was with us every step (or make that every letter) of the way. His encouragement and command of the English language were immeasurable. We are forever grateful.

Thank you, Janet Rosen, our agent, for believing in our quest and for standing behind this project from the beginning. We thank Caroline Woods, whose recommendation and introduction to Janet was pivotal. We wish to express our deepest gratitude to the tenacious Noreen Henson and the team at Demos Health Publishing, including Tom Hastings, for taking a chance on us and *The Bathroom Key*.

We feel honored to have had the opportunity to sit with Robert Kegel, Esq., and share stories about his father, Dr. Arnold Kegel. Both Kegel men are extraordinary! The generosity and grace of Donna Broderick were remarkable and most appreciated, and to the late John Broderick, Esq., may God bless you.

A pioneer's pioneer, Sean Gallagher, PT, paved the way for the world to learn from the wisdom of Joseph Pilates, and his kindness to us was unwavering. We cannot forget Valyn Carenza-Pack for her Pilates expertise and the entire staff of Praxis Physical Therapy for their enthusiasm for our project. The credit for our title goes to Elizabeth Sala, who thought of it while swimming laps with Kathryn!

Last, but certainly not least, we recognize our friends and family for their amazing support, in times of exuberance and sometimes doubt. We thank our parents for their love and for believing we could write this book. Our combined children—Denis, Gina, Jeanette (with her photographic talent), Mike (with his creative illustrations), London, and Macklin—inspire us daily in ways big and small. Finally, we thank our incredible husbands, Denes and Mark, who have wholeheartedly backed us and this project, through long nights, early mornings, and all of the places in between. We thank you all.

Introduction

WHY WE WROTE THIS BOOK

If you are tired of dealing with the untimely, embarrassing, and life-limiting challenges associated with urinary incontinence, you are holding the right book. *The Bathroom Key* will give you the knowledge, inspiration, and opportunity to rediscover an incontinence-free life. The following pages contain an effective treatment plan to successfully end your battle with incontinence, and to put you on the path toward real change.

We speak from experience, both personally and professionally. As a formerly incontinent patient, Kim has been where you are today. With Kathryn as her treating physical therapist, Kim was cured of her urinary incontinence in twelve weeks! Kim's treatment was completely natural and comprised the same physical therapy methods you will read about in this book—with no surgery, medications, or needles.

Some of you may have previously shared your incontinence issue with a friend or your physician. For others, this book is your first step toward exploring a solution. You are not alone; quite the opposite is true. You are among the estimated 200 million people suffering with incontinence worldwide. Most suffer silently. Sadly, the indignity felt by women living with urinary incontinence perpetuates the silence. The average incontinent woman waits eight years before seeking treatment. It is ironic that in a world where the reality show "Celebrity Rehab" can be followed on Twitter, and television talk shows provoke their audiences with topics like incest and erectile dysfunction, urinary incontinence is still considered taboo!

When the notion of writing this book was in its earliest stages, Kim asked friends if they had any issues with incontinence. She was amazed to learn that most of them did; however, why didn't any of them talk about it? Instead, Kim found they just accepted it as a side effect of childbirth, or something that happens with age. Kim knew from Kathryn that urinary incontinence is *not* a normal part of aging.

Kim's final epiphany came the day she watched an educational video during a physical therapy session: While the women on the video shared their triumphs in overcoming incontinence through physical therapy, they also hid their faces from the camera to protect their identities. Kim sat stunned as she recognized (and later confirmed) the voice of one of her best girlfriends on the video. Kim never knew that she and her friend shared the same struggle. This further reinforced the need for a vehicle to get people talking. The shame surrounding urinary incontinence can be so suffocating that it forces women to face the problem alone versus confiding in their friends for support.

One statement at the end of the video—that urinary incontinence is the leading cause of nursing home placement in women—drove Kim to speak with Kathryn about writing a book. Kim knew from her own experience in physical therapy that incontinence *can* be corrected. Urinary incontinence is not an indication that one needs to be placed in an assisted-living facility: Women need to be told there is another way.

As a leading physical therapist and advocate for women's health, Kathryn had already cured 4,000 incontinent women in southern California in fifteen years. Now we had to scale up! With missionary zeal, we resolved to write a book that would reach, and influence, a far greater audience. We researched the books already available on the subject and were astonished to find a gap in the marketplace. The shelves of the Women's Health section of the bookstores were devoid of anything user-friendly on incontinence. Instead, we found the shelves weighted with thick medical textbooks for nursing students and guides for caregivers. Most explained how to manage incontinent patients and seem geared toward a geriatric generation. What about the postpartum moms, or the newly menopausal? Where was the book for the everyday woman who needed answers?

Professionals at the National Institutes of Health (NIH) perfectly echoed our frustration by concluding that "coverage in popular media, advocacy from consumer groups, and reliable Internet and print material educational resources" is critically necessary to fill the knowledge gaps (Landefeld et al., 2008, p. 456). They went on to plead for more resources to bring "urinary incontinence into focus, establish it as no longer a taboo topic, and promote understanding of the isolation and impairment of daily life experienced by those affected, and encourage care seeking" (Landefeld et al., 2008, p. 456). Something needed to be done.

We thus set forth to create that book, the missing link, or "key," if you will. In this book, we share stories from other incontinent women and give you straightforward information to help you better understand your particular situation. We have included chapters on organ prolapse and pelvic pain, both of which can accompany urinary incontinence. Most important, we give you a *plan*—a comprehensive home program that will lead you to a leak-free life.

Contrary to the claims in some television ads, there is no magic pill to rid you of your incontinence. The adult diaper and personal care brands have substantially increased their marketing efforts to reach a vastly growing market. An article in the May 13, 2011, edition of *The Wall Street Journal* reported that "[Japan] will sell more adult diapers than kids diapers by 2013" (Zuckerman & Elder, 2011, p. C3). However, we refuse to let you settle by using incontinence pads as "Band-Aids", wearing them every day for the rest of your life; instead, we have a *fix*. You must work to get there, and we do not promise overnight success. The natural plan in this book is accepted mainstream medicine, and it will change your life. We are living proof. Welcome to *The Bathroom Key*.

> "All truths are easy to understand once they are discovered;
> the point is to discover them."
> —Galileo Galilei

1 The Hidden Epidemic of Urinary Incontinence

"NO LONGER A DANCING QUEEN": MEET ERICA

*A*s I turned the corner into the hotel bar, I recognized Julie immediately. We had been best friends in high school, but we hadn't seen each other in years. Tonight, we were rendezvousing with some of our old buddies for cocktails before heading over to the main ballroom for our ten-year high school reunion. I had been looking forward to this night for months. Julie and I had decided to come together, and our respective spouses were happy to be spared a night of small talk, not having attended our alma mater. Giggling together, we were as excited as two kids in a candy store.

The happy hour was lively, to say the least, as more old friends showed up to tell stories and reminisce. It was during one of these hilarious stories that I realized I was laughing so hard I was crying. The down side was that my laughter had caused a bit of leakage into my underwear. Luckily, being aware of my problem, I had worn a protective pad and had a spare tucked in my tiny clutch.

Soon, it was time to head to the ballroom. The band was already playing when our gang entered the large room, and before I knew it I was out on the dance floor grooving with my old friends. That's when it hit again, another leak, but this one was bigger than the last. Hoping everything was okay, I danced a little more, but with every move another trickle dripped out. I fled the dance floor and rushed to the bathroom. My pad was soaked. I quickly changed it and hurried back to the ballroom. Dinner was being served, so I found my table.

While I enjoyed the dinner conversation, I tried not to laugh too hard for fear I'd have another accident. After dinner my friends made their way back to the dance floor again. But I just sat and watched at the vacant table. Finally, an old boyfriend persuaded me to dance, but just like before, urine

1

would dribble onto my pad with every step I took. Nervously, I waited for the song to end and excused myself, saying that I needed a drink of water at my table. I was not enjoying myself.

When I sat down, I realized I had an even bigger problem. I could feel that my pad was so completely saturated that urine was oozing out of it. Unfortunately, I was out of fresh pads. Ashamed, I spent the rest of the reunion on my feet, but off the dance floor. I had prepped for this night for months, with a new haircut and a new dress. I had lost five pounds, yet there I stood, feeling old and disappointed. To think, I was once crowned homecoming queen. I saw it like a headline: "Former Homecoming Queen Needs Diaper to Dance at Reunion." I grimaced at my sad but true situation. I imagined what others would think if they knew of my secret condition.

Have you ever accidentally wet your pants? Like Erica, most women have. What may surprise you is how many vibrant, well-known women do it all the time. The TV anchorwoman wears adult diapers during her newscast. The New York Marathon runner has urine running down her leg and Olympic Gold Medalist Mary Lou Retton admits she leaks. Even Oscar-winning actress and mega star, Whoopi Goldberg, has publically broadcast her incontinence through an ad campaign, as well as on her popular TV show, "The View." Following suit, reality TV star, Kris Kardashian Jenner, admits that she, too, suffers with incontinence.

Urinary incontinence (the unwanted leakage of urine) has hit epidemic proportions, though for most women, it remains a hidden problem. Thirty-four million Americans live with urinary incontinence. Even more staggering is that an estimated 200 million suffer from incontinence worldwide. Over fifty percent of all women will experience incontinence at some point in their lives. To put these numbers in perspective, consider the fact that skin cancer and breast cancer are the most common forms of cancer that afflict women, yet incontinence is twenty times more prevalent than breast cancer and skin cancer combined! We will teach you how to beat these odds.

The average incontinent woman waits a shocking *eight years* to report her condition to anyone, including her own physician. The worst part is that, left untreated, incontinence can worsen until the woman is forced to spend her final years in a nursing home. The number one reason for nursing home placement among women is not senility, not lack of mobility, but incontinence. If a woman is living with one of her children, and the house starts to smell because of her incontinence, that is often the last straw leading to nursing home placement. Most of us would rather avoid this separation from our loved ones and this totally preventable scenario. This is an unacceptable final outcome for a curable medical condition.

On the island of Borneo, in Malaysia, every female teenager is taught pelvic floor exercises in preparation for marriage. The incidence of urinary incontinence in Bornean females is 1:100 versus the Western world's ratio of 1:3. In some African villages, a new mother can resume having sex only *after* she is able to give a tight vaginal squeeze around the finger of the tribal midwife. So, what do the women of Borneo and Africa know that we in the Western world do not? First, they understand the major role the pelvic floor plays in childbirth, supporting the internal organs, the sexual response, and continence. They also know that urinary incontinence is not a normal aftereffect of childbirth, menopause, or general aging.

While American teenage girls are learning how to shave their legs and download their phone photos to Facebook, the women of Africa and Borneo are learning a life lesson that will better serve their health for years to come. Our job in this book is to take the knowledge of these ancient cultures and modernize them for you through advanced physical therapy techniques.

It all starts with the pelvic floor. The pelvic floor muscles are located at the bottom (or floor) of your pelvis. They attach like a hammock from the underside of your pubic bone to your tailbone. If you are sitting as you read this book, you are sitting on your pelvic floor muscles right now. They are just under the skin, between your "sit bones." In Chapter 2 we provide illustrations of the pelvic floor muscles.

The pelvic floor muscles have two major roles in preventing incontinence. First, they function as the main sphincters that allow you to hold back urine (like tightening a faucet), yet they also allow you to urinate when you desire (like opening a faucet). Second, these important skeletal muscles support all of the abdominal organs, including the bladder. Skin alone is not strong enough to do it.

There are three openings that pass through the pelvic floor muscles in women: the urethra (for urination), the vagina (for sexual intercourse and the delivery of babies), and the rectum (for gas and bowel movements). Something strong, thick, and supportive is needed for all these important bodily functions, and the pelvic floor is designed for all these purposes.

Dr. Arnold Kegel gets credit for researching these core muscles back in the 1940s, as well as for bringing them into the limelight.

Dr. Kegel, a gynecologist practicing in southern California, found that it was incredibly difficult to teach his female incontinent patients to locate and strengthen their hidden pelvic floor muscles correctly and effectively, when they couldn't see or feel them and no joints moved when they contracted them. To overcome this, he invented and patented a pressure-sensing biofeedback unit. Voila! With his biofeedback unit, he had great success in curing urinary incontinence, and this was the basis of his published research. Without biofeedback, he failed to cure incontinence, because his verbal instructions were simply not enough.

Unfortunately, Kegel exercises, as they are called, have gotten a bad name over the years, because the term has been applied to Dr. Kegel's failure group! Lots of women try Kegel exercises and claim, "They don't work." This most likely is because they are not doing the exercises correctly. In Chapter 2 we discuss in more detail the pelvic floor, Dr. Kegel, and surface electromyographic (SEMG) biofeedback, including special techniques to make sure you locate and exercise your pelvic floor muscles correctly and effectively to prevent incontinence.

From an early age, Western women grow accustomed to wearing sanitary pads or using tampons once a month during menstruation. It is easy to reach for an absorbent pad and put a "Band-Aid" on the problem. Men can also fall victim to urinary incontinence; however, most men who become incontinent report it to their doctors right away. Men do not wear pads and do not wish to start. Men get help.

If so many women have urinary incontinence, where are they? Why don't you see them or know about them? The answer is that you do. They are your best friends, your coworkers, and potentially your sister and your mother. They are in hiding. Perhaps you haven't noticed their incontinence because their masking strategies are so well honed. It is amazing how creative we can get when covering up our incontinence. You will read examples of this throughout the book as you meet a variety of women, both young and old, currently living with incontinence. As you will learn, ignoring and concealing incontinence are not solutions; instead, those tactics just perpetuate the problem and allow it to worsen.

If there is a cure out there, why don't you know about it? In an era when every other once-closeted subject is discussed openly in the media, including yeast infections and erectile dysfunction, incontinence has remained in the dark as a private issue. Likewise, treatment for incontinence is not discussed openly. Although in recent years the Kegel exercises have become somewhat better known, this book is about much more than just Kegels. We will tell you how technological advancements (including computerized SEMG biofeedback, bladder retraining, and Pilates exercises) have produced new, noninvasive treatments for the various types of incontinence.

Worse than not talking about incontinence is the epidemic of accepting it. Too many incontinent people tolerate the condition as normal. It's not. It is not normal under any circumstance. Not normal during pregnancy. Not normal after childbirth. Not normal after menopause. Not a normal part of aging. Incontinence is *never normal*, because it is *curable*.

If you suffer with incontinence you will value this book, because it promises a radical change in the quality of your life after incontinence. However, before you can cure it, you need to understand it. What exactly is urinary incontinence, and how do you know you have it?

TYPES OF URINARY INCONTINENCE DEFINED

Using correct terminology will help you identify which type of incontinence you are dealing with and how to go about resolving it.

So, what is incontinence? Urinary incontinence is any unwanted leakage of urine. It can happen to active, healthy people of any age or gender. Incontinence is not limited to homebound or nursing home patients. Conversely, being continent is not having any unwanted urinary leakage, and this is the normal state for a person.

There are four common types of urinary incontinence: stress, urge, mixed, and nocturnal enuresis:

1. *Stress urinary incontinence:* This is the most common type of incontinence, and it is induced by physical (not mental) stress. It occurs with activity, such as coughing, sneezing, jumping, exercising, playing sports, standing up from a chair, walking, squatting, turning in bed, stair climbing, or lifting. These activities put increased pressure on the bladder, overpowering the sphincter muscles and causing leakage. We discuss stress urinary incontinence further in Chapters 2 and 3.

2. *Urge urinary incontinence:* This is leakage triggered by a strong, uncontrollable urge to immediately urinate. It typically occurs on the way to the bathroom. Triggers such as arriving home, running water, cold weather, mental stress, and worry can make urge incontinence worse. There are a few conditions related to

urge incontinence, such as frequency (multiple bathroom trips), urgency (overpowering urge), and nocturia (nighttime bathroom trips), which we discuss in more detail in Chapters 4 and 5.

3. *Mixed urinary incontinence:* In this condition, the symptoms of stress and urge urinary incontinence occur together. This is very common, and usually either stress or urge incontinence is the dominant problem.

4. *Nocturnal enuresis:* This is the medical term for bedwetting while asleep. This diagnosis applies regardless of whether protective padding is worn. It is typical for urine to seep out the leg of the diaper or pad if one is in a side-lying sleeping position, resulting in wet bed linens.

It is understandable that some women feel angry and defeated as these devastating issues negatively affect their lives. Fortunately for you, a physical therapy home treatment plan can cure all of these types of incontinence!

PROTECTIVE PADDING

Although the goal of this book is to eliminate the need to wear pads, until then, you might as well wear the right kind. Many women erroneously grab for menstrual pads, out of habit, but there are protective pads designed specifically for incontinence that hold a lot more, and they do not look like diapers. These stick-on pads for bladder control range in size from thin liners to heavy, overnight pads. The viscosity of urine is lower (thinner) than blood, so the absorbent material is engineered to hold much more urine. The top brands include Poise®, Tena Serenity®, Tranquility®, and Elyte®. Don't let the slightly higher price (compared to menstrual pads) deter you, because you will be changing less often, and you will feel more protected.

UNCOVERING COMMON MISCONCEPTIONS

Because urinary incontinence is rarely discussed openly, there are many myths and misconceptions floating around in the general public. Take the following short quiz and see what you think is true or false about this common problem.

Quiz Yourself: True or False?

Are the following statements true or false?

1. Urinary incontinence is a normal part of the aging process.
   ☐ TRUE   ☐ FALSE

2. The average bladder holds 12 ounces of urine.
   ☐ TRUE   ☐ FALSE

3. It is considered normal to use the bathroom approximately every two hours.
   ☐ TRUE   ☐ FALSE

4. If you are incontinent and planning to have more children, you can't do anything to help your incontinence until after you are finished having children.
   ☐ TRUE   ☐ FALSE

5. Drinking less will help prevent urinary incontinence.
   ☐ TRUE   ☐ FALSE

6. Women who have C-sections with every birth will not develop urinary incontinence.
   ☐ TRUE   ☐ FALSE

7. In older adults, it is normal to get up twice during the night to use the bathroom.
   ☐ TRUE   ☐ FALSE

8. Some types of beverages can cause urinary incontinence.
   ☐ TRUE   ☐ FALSE

9. Going to the bathroom more often is a good way to prevent urinary accidents.
   ☐ TRUE   ☐ FALSE

10. Professional athletes don't have urinary incontinence.
    ☐ TRUE   ☐ FALSE

The answer to Question 8 is "true." All of the other answers are "false." Here are the explanations to all ten questions:

1. Urinary incontinence is very common, but *never* normal at any age.
2. The average bladder holds 16 ounces of urine.
3. It is considered normal to urinate every three to four hours, even with good hydration. Urinating every two hours is a sign of urinary frequency.
4. You can treat your incontinence with physical therapy any time, even during pregnancy or between pregnancies.
5. Drinking less creates dark, concentrated, acidic urine that is more irritating to your bladder. Lower fluid intake could increase the risk of urge incontinence.
6. Incontinence can occur in anyone, including men, teenagers, and women who have never given birth.
7. It is normal to sleep through the night without getting up to use the bathroom. Older adults may get up once at night and still have normal bladder habits.
8. Alcoholic drinks, coffee, caffeinated tea, cola, orange juice, and grapefruit juice can irritate the bladder and make incontinence worse.
9. By the time you leave the bathroom, your kidneys have already made several more ounces of urine, so the bladder is never really empty, and leakage is always possible. Voiding too often can create a frequency problem, as the bladder "forgets" how to stretch to hold a full 16 ounces of urine.
10. It is common for runners, tennis players, golfers, and other athletes to leak urine while competing, due to a lack of strength, endurance, and coordination in their pelvic floor muscles.

Don't worry if you gave some wrong answers. Although everyone urinates, the general public gets little information about it. American sex education classes do not cover bladder health. After potty training is complete, our mothers do not sit down and teach us about adult incontinence. Chances are, unfortunately, they do not know the details themselves. Accurate information on normal bladder habits and how to retrain the bladder has not crossed over from the medical community to the public. The newly available and highly successful treatment of urinary incontinence, using physical therapy and computerized biofeedback, is still too new to be common knowledge.

Turn to the Kassai Self-Assessment for Urinary Control in Appendix I (page 243) and make three photocopies of the form. Fill one out now, to document the severity of your current incontinence, before you get underway with the treatment plans offered throughout this book. Complete the additional copies periodically, as well as when you finish the book. In Chapter 10 we provide scoring instructions that will allow you to compare future scores with this initial one. Objectively documenting your improvement will be exciting and motivating. If a physician and physical therapist are treating you, share your information with them, too.

This book will educate you about your own body, so you can take charge and overcome the common, embarrassing, underreported, and life-altering condition of incontinence. Don't let your bladder hold you captive. Instead, let this book set you (pad) free!

DISCOVERING NORMAL BLADDER FUNCTION

We humans are meant to have control over our bladders. We should empty our bladders five to seven times in a twenty-four-hour period, including zero times at night, or once for a senior citizen. Urination is one of the most common bodily functions, yet most people haven't a clue about how the process of urination takes place.

This is how it should work: The bladder is a muscle. It is called the *detrusor muscle*. When this muscle is stretched because it is filling up with urine, it contracts and creates the urge sensation. So that urge feeling is really the bladder softly contracting.

Contrary to popular belief, urges are not commands to go to the bathroom. This is just the bladder's way of drawing attention to itself, as if to say, "When it is convenient for you—and I know you are busy right now—please consider emptying me in awhile." After this mild first urge signal, it should quickly and automatically fade away without using the bathroom, allowing you to continue with whatever you were doing.

Two or three subsequent urge signals arrive and disappear, each one getting a bit stronger and with the interval between signals shrinking. Still, the actual timing of the decision to go or to wait should be up to you. You, not your bladder, should be in charge and able to delay and decide the timing of your bathroom visits. A teacher waits for class to end. A golfer waits until she arrives at the clubhouse at the end of the round. Even dogs at home wait until they are let outside. Then they go. This is the control you should have.

Normally, the final step is that you make the decision to urinate. At a time that is convenient for you, not at the demand of your bladder, you walk to the bathroom, often without even having an urge at that particular moment. Remembering all the earlier signals you were able to successfully ignore, you now consciously choose to use a coffee break at work or a commercial break in a program you are watching. Thus, *you* have chosen the time to empty your bladder on the basis of your own schedule.

Once in the bathroom, you sit on the toilet and both mentally and physically "let go." This "letting go" is what initiates the reflex to empty the bladder. What you are actually doing is letting go of the tone in your pelvic floor (Kegel) muscles. The same muscles that keep us dry are the ones that initiate the process of urination.

The brain senses the deep relaxation of your pelvic floor muscles and interprets this message as, "I want to urinate now." Actual urination may take a few seconds to begin. This is normal. The brain is busy absorbing all the sensory information available and making certain all systems are a "go." Remember, there is no rush.

Fully convinced you are ready to urinate, your brain then sends a signal down to your bladder, telling it to contract and empty. The urine flows out of your bladder, into the tube called the *urethra* and out of your body, tinkling into the toilet water. A successful void! Note that your bladder was the last participant in this process, not the first, as in the case of someone with urgency, frequency, or urge urinary incontinence.

Thus, urinating is a complex reflex involving three structures— your pelvic floor muscles, your bladder, and your brain—all working in concert to achieve perfect control:

- Your pelvic floor muscles "let go."
- Your brain perceives this "letting go" and understands that you are in the bathroom, on the toilet, and ready.
- Your brain sends a signal to your bladder that tells it to contract.
- Your bladder squeezes to empty the urine into the toilet.

Why does this process go wrong with so many women? The bladder is a very trainable organ, and it is easy for it to develop some bad habits. For these women, the bladder controls them, instead of the other way around. What do we do about it?

PHYSICAL THERAPY IS PROVEN TO END INCONTINENCE

If you are reading this book, you or someone close to you is struggling with urinary incontinence. We the authors—a former patient with urinary incontinence and the physical therapist who cured her—will give you the knowledge and the means to end your incontinence. It can be done; we are living proof.

Our intent is to free you from your incontinence and help you get important elements of your life back. We applaud you for taking this first step, for coming forward to take action against this dreaded and embarrassing condition. This book was written for you.

The good news is that there is an excellent cure for urinary incontinence. Top-notch medical journals report that physical therapy is the best treatment choice because it effectively cures the common types of incontinence. An article in the *New England Journal of Medicine* stated that physical therapy is the most desirable form of treatment for urinary incontinence (Rogers, 2008). There are no side effects to physical therapy, because it is natural and noninvasive, so a patient should try it before surgery or medications.

Professionals at the National Institutes of Health's (NIH's) 2008 state-of-the-science conference concluded that physical therapists who specialize in treating urinary incontinence (with pelvic floor muscle training and biofeedback) have successfully cured incontinence after childbirth, in older women, and in men (Landefeld et al., 2008).

That these endorsements of the physical therapy approach to incontinence come from a prestigious publication and a top-ranked national scientific group is impressive indeed.

The U.S. government has also recognized the severity of this medical issue and has made its own recommendations about treatment. The Department of Health and Human Services, Office on Women's Health, tells incontinent women to find a pelvic floor physical therapist to get treatment for their problem.

These authoritative sources are convinced that physical therapy is highly successful against the common types of incontinence. Physical therapy is mainstream medicine, and its effectiveness has been proven and recognized by the medical community. Furthermore, Medicare and most health insurance plans cover the physical therapy treatment of urinary incontinence.

A recent article in *The Los Angeles Times* reported on the widespread, hidden epidemic of urinary incontinence and how the noninvasive physical therapy approach "makes a dramatic difference in people's lives" (Schuyler, 2008).

An earlier article in *The New York Times* asserted that behavioral changes and pelvic floor exercises should be the first-line treatment for urinary incontinence; it also noted that "Doctors say the biggest battle in treating incontinence may be getting the word out so that women will seek help" (Heaner, 2005). This is the mission of *The Bathroom Key*.

You might ask, if physical therapy is so effective at curing incontinence, why didn't I already know about it and take advantage of it? Is physical therapy for incontinence still relatively new? The answer is yes. The advent of the personal computer in the 1990s brought physical therapy into focus as a viable treatment for incontinence.

Using surface electromyography (SEMG) technology connected to laptop computers, a physical therapist can show you, on a computer screen, your otherwise hidden muscles: how to find them and whether they are weak, lack endurance, or lack coordination. As mentioned earlier, these hidden muscles are located between your "sit bones," in the floor of your pelvis, and they are responsible for keeping you continent. Augmented by the SEMG biofeedback machine, with stick-on electrodes, you can actually *see* these muscles working on the computer screen. This SEMG biofeedback technique is totally painless and noninvasive. There are no needles and no electric shock whatsoever. The experience is quite similar to what one sees and feels with an electrocardiogram (EKG), because both devices graphically record muscle contractions.

Without this new technology, it is quite impossible to rehabilitate a muscle that is invisible, too weak to feel, and doesn't move any joint. The SEMG biofeedback approach is a natural one directed at the root cause of the problem: pelvic floor muscle weakness. Through bladder retraining, the same muscles are used to regain control of an overactive bladder, without medications. Depending on the severity of the incontinence, the duration of physical therapy treatment usually ranges from eight to sixteen visits, generally once a week. The patient's home treatment plan is initiated on the first visit and progresses throughout the course of physical therapy. The home program you will learn about in this book will follow a similar timetable.

THE TREATMENT PLAN TO NATURALLY CURE YOUR INCONTINENCE

The physical therapy method to end your incontinence involves no surgery, no medications, and no needles. It is mainstream medicine that offers you a proven program to get cured. Natural behavioral methods are coupled with a precise recipe of targeted exercises to rid you of your embarrassing and annoying incontinence. Physical therapy does not treat symptoms with masking techniques; instead, it gets to the underlying cause of the problem and provides a formula that *works*!

Why not cure your incontinence by simply addressing the underlying causes—namely, pelvic floor weakness and an overactive bladder? The physical therapy treatment plan discussed in this book will put you on the road to recovery in a matter of weeks. How long have you been incontinent? How much longer do you want to wait to be cured?

The National Institutes of Health (NIH) fully supports the physical therapy approach (Landefeld et al., 2008). Its recommendations have been thoroughly reviewed by scientific experts, who concluded that physical therapy can cure incontinence: "Women with bladder control problems can regain control through pelvic muscle exercises." This means you! The NIH also encourages women to seek professional help to make sure they are exercising the right muscles. You have taken that first step by reading this book.

The NIH has made its literature on this subject readily available to the public. By intentionally not copyrighting its Internet pamphlet, it "encourages users of this publication to duplicate and distribute as many copies as desired." Our government wants this vital information to be disseminated as common knowledge, and the program in this book will accomplish exactly this. Share your experience with a friend and pass along the secret of *The Bathroom Key*.

Equipped with this new information to fight incontinence, you are destined for success. Outlined next are the eleven comprehensive elements of the home program you will implement, which will become your bathroom key, freeing you from the domination of your bladder:

1. Your Home Program to Find Your Pelvic Floor
2. Your Home Program for Stress Urinary Incontinence

3. Your Home Program to Prevent Urinary Tract Infections
4. Your Home Program: How to Complete a Voiding Diary
5. Your Home Program: How to Retrain Your Bladder
6. Your Home Program for Urge Suppression Techniques
7. Your Home Program for Dietary Substitutions and Hydration
8. Your Home Program with Mat Pilates
9. Your Home Program for Organ Prolapse
10. Your Home Program for Pelvic Pain and Sexual Issues
11. Your Home Program to Regain the Joy in Your Life

If more women knew that such a powerful, natural cure through physical therapy is available, they wouldn't be so concerned about concealing their incontinence. Urologist Liao Limin of the Chinese Urological Association reported that "About 24% to 45% of women in the world have had urinary incontinence problems at least once in their lives (after reaching the age of 18)" (quoted in Wanli, 2010). *The Wall Street Journal* recently reported that "[Japan] will sell more adult diapers than kids diapers by 2013" (Zuckerman & Eder, 2011, p. C3). It is our sincere hope that this prediction does not come true. It doesn't have to. In August 2011, the leading health article on Oprah.com affirmed that "with proper strengthening, the data shows there's an 85 percent chance of complete resolution [of urinary incontinence]," according to Jennifer Klestinski, MPT, Communications Director of the Women's Health Section of the American Physical Therapy Association (Pikul, 2011).

This book is aimed at getting the word to the estimated 200 million incontinent adults worldwide. Physical therapy is the genuine answer to their bathroom woes and, thankfully, much of it can be done at home.

> "The road to success is always under construction."
> —Lily Tomlin

2 Stress Urinary Incontinence

"LICKED HER PROBLEM": MEET TERRY

*M*y urinary incontinence started eleven years ago. I can even pinpoint the date, because it coincides with the birth of my third child. After my first two kids were born, I was just fine. But it was the birth of my third and final baby, Michael, that seemed to cause me the most distress. After that delivery, I have never been the same. It seemed to take my body a lot longer to get back into shape than it had with my first two kids, and I still had a nagging feeling of instability in my midsection.

My maternity leave seemed to fly by, and soon it was time to return to work. My career has always been very important to me, and I am passionate about it. I love the balance it brings to my life as a mother. I have worked in the fashion industry since I graduated from college. Through the years, I have represented various designers, selling their lines to large department stores and boutiques. This career is ideal for me, because I love fashion and interacting with people.

I had a beautiful new suit I had been hoping to wear on my first day back to work, and I was thrilled when it fit! It was a lovely periwinkle blue that I picked out before Michael was born, but now I wore it in honor of my wonderful new baby boy. I put on my favorite pair of patent leather heels, traded in my bulky diaper bag for my Coach tote, and was off.

My first day back was going well, and my coworkers had planned a "welcome back" luncheon for me in the office. We sat around the large conference table eating chicken salad, drinking buckets of iced tea, and catching up. It was great. It felt so good to be back.

Soon it was time to get back to my desk and earn my keep. I stood up, and a large spritz shot into my underwear. I quickly sat down again and tried to act nonchalant. These ladies were some of my best friends. I had worked with them for years, but still I could not bring myself to tell anyone

15

about my hidden problem. Instead I waited until, one by one, my cowork-
ers left the conference room. I lingered as long as I could and then hurried
to my office. After locking the door, I quickly changed out of my gorgeous
light blue pants, which had turned dark blue through the crotch and back-
side. I began searching for an answer to this crisis.

I always had a ton of sample designs hanging in my office, but sud-
denly I wasn't sure of what was left on my rack, because I had been out
of my office for the past several months. Luckily, there was a pair of our
"around the world" pants in black. They were marketed with this name be-
cause they could literally be rolled into a ball and packed tightly in any type
of bag and still unroll looking fabulous. The fabric was a stretchy crepe, and
they were cut with a wide leg that gave them an elegant look. Those pants
fit me well enough and the black color coordinated with my blue jacket. I
was quite proud of my resourcefulness.

Once the immediacy of the problem was resolved, I started thinking
about the future. Was this going to happen again? I decided it probably
would. Would I ever get to wear pretty colors again or would I be plagued
to wear black forever? I was in the fashion industry, for goodness' sake.
Part of my job requirement was to wear the line—and the items were not
always black.

I decided to do a little test. I looked down at the new pair of pants I was
wearing, and I poured a dribble of water from the bottle on my desk onto
the pant leg. The color barely changed. These pants were available in three
other colors: cherry, stone (a light gray), and midnight. All three colors
were on the rack in my office. I grabbed my water bottle and performed
my test on each of them. Miraculously, there was little change, even to the
stone pair. I made a mental note to find out more about this fabric, and I
got back to work.

The test I did that day in my office became a standard for me. I found
many other colors and fabrics that didn't really change too much if they
got wet. Once, when I was in a dressing room trying on pants and a skirt,
I realized I didn't have any water with me. To conduct my new "test," I
licked the hem of each garment. I giggled while doing it: If anyone saw
what I was doing, she would think I had lost my mind. But my licking test
worked. Now I use this technique anytime I don't have bottled water with
me. Choosing my fabrics carefully, to handle my infrequent accidents, beats
wearing those annoying pads every day.

Although I am not happy about my incontinence, I feel a bit trium-
phant in my method of camouflaging it. I have been pouring water on or
licking my clothes for the past eleven years. It's an odd routine, I know, but
it works, and any accident I have isn't obvious to anyone but me.

Terry has the most common form of urinary incontinence: *stress urinary incontinence*, which is caused when the pelvic floor muscles are not strong enough to withstand physical strain. In Terry's case, the motion of standing up from a chair was more than her pelvic floor muscles could take. The fact that she had just drank caffeinated tea, a major bladder irritant, did not help. (See Chapter 5 for our discussion of a dietary and hydration plan to help treat incontinence.)

In addition, Terry was just back to work from her maternity leave, having endured a third pregnancy and a difficult delivery. When the pelvic floor muscles are stretched and weakened through the trauma of giving birth, even the simplest of tasks strains them.

Is Terry doomed? Of course not, but she must address her problem now. If left ignored, chances are Terry's muscles will get weaker and her spritzes larger.

Sadly, after years of neglect, incontinence can worsen, subtly and insidiously, beyond the stage at which it is controllable. As we mentioned in Chapter 1, some incontinent women wind up living in a convalescent home.

Erica, in Chapter 1, suffers from stress urinary incontinence as well. Her pelvic floor could not withstand the physical strain of laughing and dancing. You can bet jumping rope or kickboxing would prove catastrophic for either of these two ladies! Obviously, not everyone needs to jump rope, but all of us would like to laugh with friends, lunch in confidence, and maybe even do a little dancing. Read on and discover the plan that will get you living the life you want without the embarrassment of the spritz.

DO I HAVE STRESS URINARY INCONTINENCE?

Do you have stress urinary incontinence, like Terry and Erica? Let's find out so you can get your treatment plan underway! Knowing what condition you have is the first step in fixing it.

Stress urinary incontinence is defined as the accidental leakage of urine—not into the toilet—triggered by physical activity. Stress incontinence is not confined to nursing home patients. All around the world, active, vibrant women like you have this problem. Remember, "active" does not necessarily mean "athletic." As in Terry's case, the movement that caused her problem was a simple one: standing up. If you are ready to start moving again, to get rid of your pads and the associated cost and potential embarrassment, read on and get cured!

In stress incontinence it is physical stress, not mental stress, that triggers urine leakage. Look over the following partial list of very common physical activities that cause leakage in millions of women. If you have urinary leakage (however small) into your underwear with any of these activities, you have stress urinary incontinence.

Do You Accidentally Leak Urine When You Are:

Coughing?
Sneezing?
Laughing?
Blowing your nose?
Walking up or down stairs?
Exercising?
Walking?
Running?
Jumping?
Playing sports?
Lifting?
Squatting?
Standing up from a chair?
Lying down onto or getting up out of bed?
Turning in bed?
Sick with a cold or flu?
About to begin your menstrual period?

If you answered "yes" to any of these questions, this chapter can help you by giving you the treatment plan you need to get rid of this embarrassing problem. Maybe only a little bubble of urine escapes into your underwear once a month and you don't even need to wear pads, or you get your annual cold and the resultant coughing causes leakage and several underwear changes throughout the day. Perhaps you have been experiencing saturating leakage and have been changing your thick diapers for years. Regardless of whether the amount of leakage is a little or a lot, the fact is that you have stress urinary incontinence. This will not happen to you much longer, because now you have a proven plan to end your incontinence for good.

If you answered "no" to all of the questions on the list, but you still have urine leakage, then you most likely have the second most common form of urinary incontinence, called ***urge urinary*** *incontinence.* Don't be tempted to skip ahead to Chapters 4 and 5, because you must first possess adequate physical strength and endurance in your pelvic floor before you can use the material in those chapters to help treat your urge incontinence.

Many women have both stress and urge incontinence; this is termed *mixed urinary incontinence.* This is not a third kind of incontinence; it is a condition in which both stress and urge incontinence occur together. Usually one or the other—stress or urge incontinence—is the more dominant condition, but in some women they are equally problematic.

To find out which type of incontinence is your primary condition, ask yourself the following two questions:

1. Does most of my leakage happen when I am doing an activity like those in the list just provided? (This indicates that stress incontinence is primary.)

OR

2. Does most of my leakage happen when I am on my way to the bathroom, feeling the urge to go but not making it in time? (This indicates that urge incontinence is primary.)

OK. Now you know what it's called, but *why* do you have stress urinary incontinence in the first place?

Although it may seem to "run in your family" (pun intended), stress urinary incontinence is *not* a genetic condition. The mere fact that your mother, your sister, and your daughters all have urinary leakage does *not* mean the problem is hereditary. You would never say that the common cold runs in your family, yet urinary incontinence is nearly as common. Luckily, unlike the common cold, stress urinary incontinence is very curable!

WHAT CAUSES STRESS URINARY INCONTINENCE?

Weakness of your pelvic floor muscles is the culprit. These skeletal muscles (described in more detail shortly) lie at the very bottom of your pelvis. They are hidden under all of your organs.

Please try this. Look down toward your pubic bone, imagine that all of your organs are not there, and the image on the next page is what you would see.

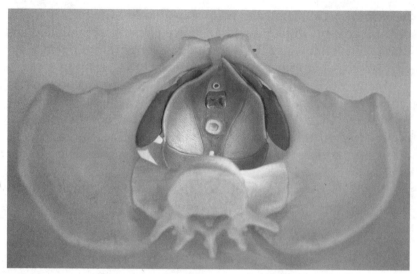

**Model of female pelvic floor muscles,
looking down into the pelvis from the head.**

"Wow!" you might exclaim. You probably never knew you *had* muscles down there. Well, you do, and those muscles do many wonderful things, the most important of which (for our purposes) is preventing urinary leakage—*if* those muscles are sufficiently strong. That is the goal of our treatment plan: to make these muscles strong enough that even when you cough, sneeze, or exercise, the urine will stay in your bladder where it belongs, until *you* choose to empty it!

Pelvic floor muscles are skeletal muscles; they are attached to your bones, just like the muscles in your arms (e.g., the biceps) and legs (e.g., the calf muscles). You should (and *can*) have voluntary control of all three of these muscle groups. Yes, you can control your pelvic floor muscles. However, there is a huge distinction between your pelvic floor muscles and the other types of muscles in your body: Both your biceps and calf muscles give you motion (e.g., the biceps muscle bends your elbow, and the calf muscle allows you to rise up onto your toes); conversely, the pelvic floor muscles give you no motion whatsoever. They do not make any part of the skeleton move. So why do you have them? The answer to that question is because they have a few other jobs to do.

The biggest role of the pelvic floor muscles (pertinent to this chapter) is that they act as a sphincter—like a faucet—to give you control of urination. When you are about to urinate and you "let go," these are the muscles you open, allowing urine to start falling out of your body through the tube called your *urethra*.

If these pelvic floor muscles are strong enough, no amount of physical activity will cause urine to leak without your consent. However, if bladder pressure exceeds the strength of your pelvic floor muscles, urine will leak. The pelvic floor must be able to successfully counteract the pressure you put on your bladder every time you lift your laundry basket, squat down to pull weeds in your garden, or go for a run in the park.

Scientists would call this a *pressure gradient*, whereby two pressure systems oppose each other and only one can win. If you stay dry when you laugh or cough, then your pelvic floor muscles won. If you leak when you blow your nose or jump, then the bladder pressure won. This is why urine does not leak all the time. When you are lying down or sitting, your leakage is probably nonexistent or rare. Very little pressure is put on your bladder when you are in the sitting or lying positions. No pressure *on* your bladder means no leakage *from* your bladder; however, changing positions can create considerable pressure on your bladder, and that pressure can and frequently does cause leakage.

Some women have had a leakage problem for years, even during childhood; however, the typical woman suffering from incontinence today had no problem at all as a child. She was able to run, bounce on a trampoline, jump down from trees, and giggle without a single leak. So, what happened? There are many answers to this question. The first conclusion you might come to is "age." This is incorrect. Urinary incontinence is *not* a normal part of the aging process.

Your second thought may be that it's due to pregnancy or childbirth. While these are leading causes of incontinence, a new study reveals that women who have never been pregnant are incontinent, too. This Australian study is the first of its kind and

> was undertaken to determine the prevalence of UI [urinary incontinence] in otherwise healthy young women aged 16 to 30 years who have never been pregnant. The research showed that 12.6 per cent of surveyed women had urinary incontinence, with most experiencing stress incontinence (6.2 per cent) or urge incontinence (4.5 per cent). About 1.9 per cent of those surveyed experienced both [mixed incontinence]. (Monash University, 2011)

The following are four of the leading causes of incontinence, due to a weakened pelvic floor:

1. *Pregnancy:* During pregnancy, the pelvic floor muscles have to support the heavier uterus and the developing fetus. Naturally, the muscles get fatigued as the pregnancy advances, just like the legs and back do. Urinary incontinence is often the result of this added burden on the pelvic floor.
2. *Childbirth:* During the birthing process, the pelvic floor is stretched to the maximum to allow the baby's head and shoulders to pass through the vaginal opening. This is called *stretch trauma*. Often, the pelvic floor muscles are actually torn during the birth, or the doctor may cut these muscles (a procedure called an *episiotomy*). Unless the pelvic floor is fully rehabilitated after giving birth, incontinence may result and linger for decades.
3. *Menopause:* The hormonal changes our bodies go through during menopause can cause a myriad of ailments, one of which is muscle weakness. When this weakness affects the pelvic floor, urinary incontinence is the unwanted symptom. Studies clearly demonstrate that, at *any* age, exercise can improve muscle strength.
4. *Immobility:* Muscle inactivity, for any reason, will lead to atrophy and muscle weakness. Anyone who has had an arm cast will surely remember how much smaller his or her arm was when the cast came off after just six weeks or so. The pelvic floor acts the same way if it is ignored and not challenged through daily exercise. It gets thin and weak and doesn't do its job of preventing incontinence.

In this chapter, we show you how to find these hidden muscles and enlighten you on the marvels of biofeedback. In Chapter 3 we give you a concrete treatment plan to overcome your stress urinary incontinence so you win the pressure gradient war. Before long, you will have the strength, endurance, and tone to stay dry, day and night.

Stress urinary incontinence has been around for ages. Nonsurgical, natural, behavioral treatment (using biofeedback and exercise) for stress urinary incontinence dates back to the 1940s. *Biofeedback* is a learning technique that uses specialized equipment to help a person gain control of bodily functions. It involves the monitoring of a life process ("bio") and the return of that information to the patient and therapist in a meaningful form ("feedback"). We now provide a little history lesson from Dr. Arnold Kegel, the founding father of the original treatment plan to cure stress urinary incontinence.

ARNOLD KEGEL, MD, AND THE PELVIC FLOOR MUSCLES

You have probably heard of *Kegel exercises*; perhaps you have even tried them. Can you do them correctly? As you read this chapter, you will learn why the Kegels you have attempted may not have been as successful as their namesake once intended. That's right: Few people realize that the name *Kegel* comes from a real man, a physician who was an amazing pioneer in the field of Women's Health.

The son of a minister, Dr. Arnold Henry Kegel (pronounced *KAY-gull*), was born in Lennox, South Dakota, in 1894 (see below image). He studied medicine at the University of Illinois and received his medical degree in 1916 (image on the next page). Although later his name became synonymous with pelvic floor exercise, gynecology was not his first passion; he was originally trained as a surgeon. With Dr. Mayo as his mentor, he studied at the world-renowned Mayo Clinic from 1917 through 1921. His surgical specialty was performing thyroidectomies for the treatment of neck goiters. At that time, the Mayo Clinic performed about 3,000 such surgeries each year, because doctors did not yet know that iodine deficiency caused goiters.

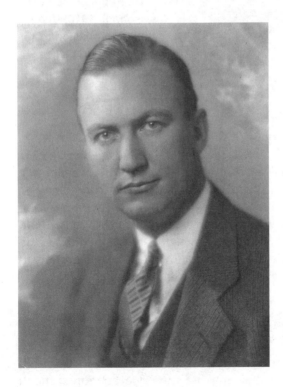

**Arnold Kegel, MD.
Used with permission
from John and Donna
Broderick.**

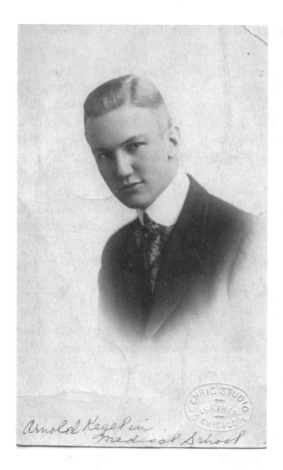

Arnold Kegel in medical school

Dr. Kegel in medical school, 1916. Used with permission from John and Donna Broderick.

In 1927, at the beckoning of the mayor of Chicago, Dr. Kegel became that city's Commissioner of Health (see image on page 25). An outbreak of an infectious disease had swept through a Chicago hospital, and no one could decipher its source. After conducting an investigation, Kegel realized that a faulty plumbing system was to blame. Kegel continued as Commissioner for the next five years and faced many challenges in Chicago during his reign, including Prohibition. He was dedicated to public health and believed strongly in the merits of compulsory vaccination of schoolchildren.

In 1935, Dr. Kegel moved to Los Angeles. He continued to perform thyroidectomies for several more years, but he was forced to take several extended breaks from surgery because of severe hand allergies to surgical gloves (R. Kegel, personal communication, March 10, 2011). In addition, symptoms from a childhood fracture to his left elbow got progressively worse, making surgery even more difficult

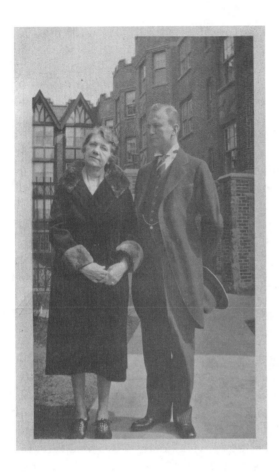

Dr. Kegel with his mother, as Health Commissioner of Chicago, circa the late 1920s. Used with permission from John and Donna Broderick.

to perform. In 1924, the Morton Salt Company began distributing iodized salt nationally, thereby halting new cases of goiters, and the need for thyroidectomies diminished. All three factors contributed to the cessation of his surgical career, and he began searching for a new focus for his medical practice.

About that time, Dr. Kegel became aware of the contractibility of the pelvic floor muscles around the vagina. He wanted to learn more about these muscles, their movement, their anatomical position, and their function, as they related to sexual issues and incontinence. According to his son Robert, Dr. Kegel took *moulage* molds (similar to dental molds) of the vaginas of living women. He discovered that live pelvic floor muscles were positioned much higher in the pelvis than was previously thought to be the case, based on cadaver dissection alone.

Dr. Kegel hypothesized that if these muscles could squeeze and contract, they could be trained and strengthened. By the late 1940s, he had found his new calling, and he concentrated on the nonsurgical approaches to gynecological problems, in particular urinary incontinence.

As an Assistant Professor of Gynecology at the University of Southern California School of Medicine in Los Angeles, Dr. Kegel published his first article in 1948, which described his new technique for training of the pelvic floor muscles. He called his new approach *physiologic therapy*, and it was a precursor to modern physical therapy treatment for incontinence (Kegel, 1951). Dr. Kegel is indisputably regarded as the founding father of the noninvasive treatment plan for urinary incontinence in women.

In 1940, skirts were long and standards were high. It took a lot of gumption for women to share their most intimate problem with their doctors, who almost invariably were male. The median age at which women married in 1940 was 21.5 years, and most were housewives. Single women made up only a fraction of the workforce. Birth control literature was still being classified as "obscene" in court cases. Heck, it had only been twenty years since Congress had passed the Nineteenth Amendment, allowing women the right to vote!

Let's put Dr. Kegel's early work in proper perspective. In the twenty-first century, television programs like "Sex and the City" break down old-fashioned barriers and discuss subjects of a very personal nature. Today's talk show hosts broadcast stories of incest and discuss impotence openly. Still, in this day and age urinary incontinence remains a taboo topic, even among girlfriends. Do you know that the average modern woman suffers for years with incontinence before she even mentions it to her physician? Imagine how it must have been for Dr. Kegel's patients nearly seventy years ago!

During World War II, however, the role of women took a new turn. Suddenly they were needed to replace men in the workplace, and women became an integral part of the war effort. Medicine was advancing as well, and in 1941 the first successful use of the antibiotic penicillin revolutionized medicine. And a doctor named Kegel was doing some pretty remarkable work, too.

Professionally, Dr. Kegel was breaking new ground, and he was doing it without the support of many of his colleagues. Other doctors of that era thought that what Dr. Kegel was doing was a waste of time. They were surgeons, and the way surgeons fixed problems was with surgery! Dr. Kegel felt differently. A "Lone Ranger" of sorts, Dr. Kegel continued his quest to help women naturally and noninvasively.

In his new gynecological practice, Dr. Kegel found urinary incontinence to be a very common complaint. As part of his evaluation of female patients, he tested the strength of their pelvic floor muscles. He found that only about sixty percent of them could achieve normal muscle contractions. "In more than 30% of women, however, no contractions, or only weak or delayed contractions, can be elicited in spite of diligent efforts," he reported (Kegel, 1951, pp. 915–917). This early research mirrors the estimated current incidence of urinary incontinence: One in three women suffers from a weak pelvic floor, which leads to urinary incontinence.

Dr. Kegel turned his attention to 300 of his incontinent female patients and noted atrophy (sagging and thinning) of the pelvic floor muscles in *all* of them. To help them, he consulted seven then-current textbooks on obstetrics and gynecology. All the books "failed to reveal any mention of active exercises for the relief of urinary stress incontinence" (Kegel, 1951, pp. 915–917). His mission continued when he unlocked the door, so to speak, and discovered the key between incontinence and pelvic floor weakness. Armed with his new theory, he was more determined than ever to develop appropriate exercises for the pelvic floor to cure incontinence.

Dr. Kegel's next hurdle was what to do about this brainstorm. In his clinical experience, "ordinarily it proved difficult to teach women with incapacitating urinary stress incontinence awareness of the (pelvic floor) muscle, and in some instances various methods of instruction had to be employed over a year's time before voluntary contractions of the muscle could be established" (Dr. Kegel, 1951, pp. 915–917). A year's time was much too long for Dr. Kegel and his patients. He was frustrated at his inability to exercise these hidden, weak, and dormant muscles with verbal instruction alone. In comparison, it is easy to train the biceps: All you need to do is hold a weight and bend the elbow. Exercising the pelvic floor muscles is not so easy, because you can't see them, can't feel them, and they don't move any joint. His search for a resolution continued.

To complicate matters, Dr. Kegel found that his patients would "invariably try to substitute contractions of extraneous muscles, especially those of the abdominal wall and gluteal region" (1951, pp. 915–917). In other words, instead of exercising the correct pelvic floor muscles, they were contracting the *wrong* muscles: in the tummy, buttocks, and inner thighs. This compounded his frustration in not being able to help his patients, because they were not making their pelvic floor muscles stronger with their incorrect and ineffective exercise technique.

After years of persistent research, Dr. Kegel invented a device that would forever change the way he treated his incontinent patients. He designed a pressure sensor (an air-filled tube) that he inserted vaginally. His patients squeezed the device using their pelvic floor muscles, enabling them at last to find, observe, and exercise these important muscles. Even better, Dr. Kegel had attached a pressure gauge, which allowed him to measure and record how hard each patient could squeeze her pelvic floor muscles. He used the same cues we use today: Squeeze as if to hold back gas or a bowel movement, clamp around the vagina, or pretend you are trying to stop the urine flow.

Dr. Kegel was advanced in his thinking when he wrote, "It is necessary to establish a connection between contractions of the [pelvic floor] and the sense of sight" (Kegel, 1948a). Without an eye-to-muscle connection, he had failed to cure incontinence. However, with his new biofeedback device, the Kegel Perineometer (pronounced *per-eh-knee-AHM-eh-ter*), he was finally able to help his patients make that connection.

The Kegel Perineometer was awarded a U.S. patent in 1951 and is pictured on the next page. Large corporate investment in medical devices was not commonplace in the early 1950s, so the device was sold on a relatively small scale. Nevertheless, the importance of biofeedback in educating and training women on their pelvic floors was solidified.

The Kegel Perineometer was the first biofeedback device invented for the pelvic floor muscles, and it allowed women to actually *see* their pelvic floor muscles at work. This was a dramatic development in the field! Frankly, over the past seven decades, this biofeedback concept has restored the lives of countless incontinent women worldwide. Thank you, Dr. Kegel!

Dr. Kegel used the device for training as well. He could control the amount of air in the chamber, offering gentle resistance to the muscle and making it stronger and stronger as the incontinence melted away (Kegel, 1948b). Training with the Perineometer encouraged the women to do *better* each time, by exerting more *measurable* pressure with their muscle contractions. That made his patients' success rate skyrocket. Using his Perineometer and physiologic therapy on 500 patients, he restored continence in eighty-four percent of them (Kegel, 1951). His verbal instructions had failed, but his new biofeedback device had succeeded!

For nearly seventy years, people have been using the term *Kegel exercise* to mean any exercise of the pelvic floor muscles. This has given Kegel exercises a reputation for being unsuccessful, when in fact verbal instruction alone did not work for Dr. Kegel himself,

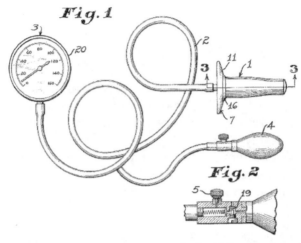

Feb. 13, 1951   A. H. KEGEL   2,541,520

METHOD AND APPARATUS TO INDICATE OR OBSERVE
PROGRESSIVE EXERCISE OF INJURED
SPHINCTER MUSCLES
Filed Jan. 13, 1947

Dr. Kegel's Perineometer was awarded a U.S. patent in 1951.

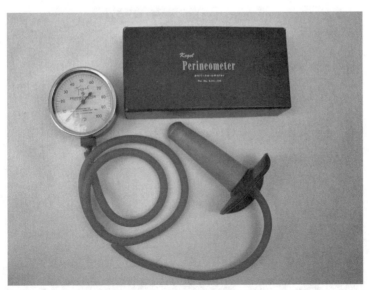

Dr. Kegel's original biofeedback device, called the Perineometer.

either! Without the benefit of biofeedback, most women are unable to do the exercises correctly. Dr. Kegel's monumental contribution was his identification of the necessity of biofeedback to identify and exercise the pelvic floor muscles to cure incontinence, yet most people do not know that. As a matter of fact, physical therapy purists say that only when a woman is connected to a biofeedback unit is she truly doing a Kegel exercise.

Dr. Kegel's dedication to his patients and his relentless drive to cure them made him a hero to many people, including us authors and all physical therapists who specialize in pelvic floor rehabilitation. Dr. Kegel needed biofeedback to find and train this muscle, and you probably do, too. But don't worry; you will be taught ways you can benefit from the various types of biofeedback later in this chapter. Biofeedback of some variety should be an integral part of every treatment plan to alleviate incontinence.

INTRODUCING SURFACE ELECTROMYOGRAM (SEMG) BIOFEEDBACK

Today, the advent of the laptop computer has taken Dr. Kegel's principles of biofeedback to a more sophisticated level. Computerized

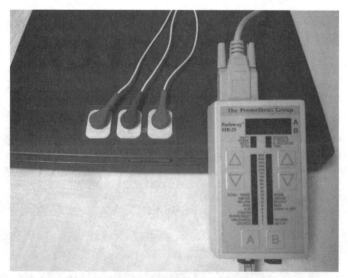

Modern computerized SEMG biofeedback device (by The Prometheus Group) with stick-on electrodes.

surface electromyogram (SEMG) units have replaced the Kegel Perineometer (see opposite page).

Doctors use needles when they perform EMGs (electromyograms). Luckily for incontinent women, physical therapists use no needles. SEMG usually involves stick-on electrodes placed on the buttocks. SEMG biofeedback is totally noninvasive and involves no electrical shock or "zapping" whatsoever! The electrodes merely record the electricity the pelvic floor muscles put out.

SEMG units work very similar to the way electrocardiograms (EKGs) work for the heart. You may not have known this, but every muscle in the body puts out electricity, not just the heart muscle. Whereas an EKG records the electrical activity of the heart muscle, SEMG biofeedback records the electrical activity of the pelvic floor muscles. Both the EKG and the SEMG machines provide graphic representations of this electricity. Everyone is familiar with an EKG graph, either from personal experience or from watching any medical TV show. The SEMG graph is similar.

The SEMG device measures the amount of electricity coming from the pelvic floor as its muscles contract. The harder the muscles are squeezed, the higher the graph climbs, forming a jagged peak. The typical patient is excited to actually *see* her hidden and weak pelvic floor muscles at work. She makes the connection that Dr. Kegel knew was so important—namely, what she feels in her muscles is perfectly reinforced by what she sees on the computer screen.

But where do the electrodes go? Two stick-on electrodes are placed alongside your "sit bones" (called the *ischial tuberosities*), on the skin over the pelvic floor muscles. These are the two bones you feel when you sit on hard bleachers at a sporting event. Please note that SEMG is entirely different from the electrical stimulation treatment commonly used in physical therapy clinics or athletic training rooms. The woman does not feel any electricity whatsoever coming from the electrodes, and the machine causes no muscles to twitch. Just like during an EKG, you feel nothing.

As you can see on page 32, modesty and comfort are preserved as physical therapist/coauthor Kathryn Kassai performs an actual SEMG biofeedback session with coauthor and formerly incontinent patient Kim Perelli.

Kim feels no electricity as she sits on three small stick-on electrodes. She is fully clothed and comfortably seated with the SEMG wires coming out of her waistband as she trains her pelvic floor muscles on the computer. Most women's first reaction when they see

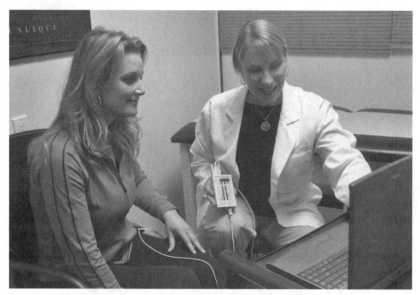

An actual SEMG biofeedback session taking place.
Left: Author Kim Perelli (a former patient).
Right: Author Kathryn Kassai, Kim's physical therapist.

their pelvic floor muscles working and displayed on the computer screen is, "WOW, this is so cool! Now I *know* I am doing it right!"

How excited would Dr. Kegel have been if *he* had this technology? Every little twitch of the pelvic floor muscles is recorded on a graph that lets the patient *see* her muscles working as she *feels* them working. This colorful graph, created by the computer, makes it obvious how well (or how poorly) the muscles are working, which in turn helps the woman work even harder.

The next page shows an actual SEMG graph of Kim's pelvic floor muscles as she squeezes them eight times. Can you see that she started getting a little tired on the fourth contraction? Over the course of several physical therapy sessions, the SEMG biofeedback encourages her to make stronger contractions. You can easily see that the peak in Kim's graph, as seen on the second graph on the next page, is now much higher, because she is giving a harder squeeze that produces more electricity. Kim's home exercise program succeeded in making her pelvic floor stronger, and you will learn a program of your own in Chapter 3. Her stronger contractions were also due to the motivational factor of being able to see exactly what is going on with this hidden muscle and naturally wanting to do better

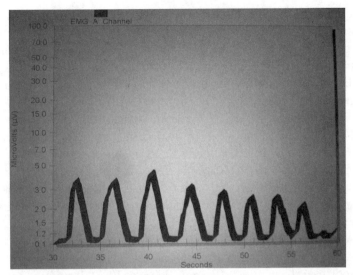

Kim's computerized SEMG biofeedback graphs, depicting eight
contractions, showing fatigue on the fourth contraction.

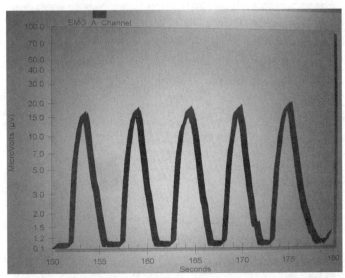

Kim's computerized SEMG biofeedback graphs, showing five
contractions with much better strength.

and better. It was quite inspirational when Kathryn compared Kim's current graphs with her initial graphs that were produced on her first physical therapy visit. Every woman loves to see the results of her hard efforts shown objectively on the computer. Of course, the real benefit is a gradual lessening of incontinence, with fewer and smaller urine leaks.

Computerized SEMG is far more sensitive and accurate than the Kegel Perineometer was in evaluating, identifying, and rehabilitating weak or injured pelvic floor muscles. Today, pelvic floor muscle training with SEMG biofeedback is the gold standard in any treatment plan to overcome incontinence. Pelvic floor exercises— using biofeedback—are highly regarded as the first-line treatment for stress urinary incontinence.

A recent study published in the *New England Journal of Medicine* noted that the "first-line treatment for stress incontinence includes pelvic floor muscle training" (Rogers, 2008, p. 1031). It pointed out that women unable to identify their pelvic floor muscles "may benefit from seeing a physical therapist trained in pelvic floor therapy" (Rogers, 2008, p. 1031). Note that only physical therapists who specialize in the treatment of incontinence (or "Women's Health," as it is also called) will have computerized SEMG equipment for inclusion in an individualized treatment plan. Consult Appendix III on page 247 to find one.

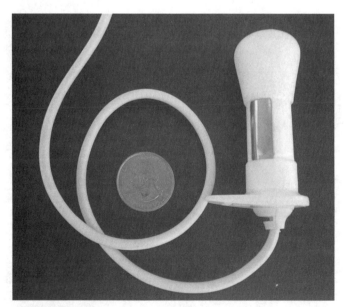

An SEMG vaginal sensor, used in special cases only.

In special cases, when the muscles are nearly dormant, the physical therapist may opt to use a vaginal sensor that looks like a small tampon in order to get closer to the pelvic floor muscle (see opposite). Don't worry—the patient still feels no electricity. The vaginal sensor works the same way as a stick-on electrode, and it is only "listening" to the muscle and recording its electrical impulses.

What if you don't have access to physical therapy, or you want to try to see what you can do on your own first? We will certainly show you how to do that. In the next section we discuss some low-tech ways to locate and train your pelvic floor muscles. After all, a home exercise program is a mandatory part of every treatment plan for incontinence, with or without SEMG biofeedback.

YOUR HOME PROGRAM TO FIND YOUR PELVIC FLOOR

The best way to identify your pelvic floor muscles is to go to a licensed physical therapist who specializes in treating incontinence and have him or her perform SEMG biofeedback; however, there are other ways to locate them successfully. In this section we teach you four ways to locate them at home, so you'll know that you will be exercising the correct muscles in your home treatment plan, which we present in the next chapter.

The image on the next page provides a different view of your pelvic floor muscles. The angle is taken from the opposite direction as the one earlier in this chapter. If you are lying on your back with your legs open (picture the position you would assume for your annual pap smear test), and your skin was removed, this is what you would see. Like most skeletal muscles, these muscles are right below the skin. They are close to the outside of you, not "way up inside" as many women think.

Can you locate the four structures that pierce right through these muscles? The pelvic floor muscles control the function of all four. From top (below your pubic bone) to bottom (above your tailbone), the following four structures pass right through your pelvic floor muscles:

1. Clitoris: the nodule below the pubic bone that is a sex organ
2. Urethra: the tiny hole where urine comes out
3. Vagina: the larger opening, for sexual intercourse and giving birth
4. Rectum: the thick circular muscle where gas and bowel movements exit

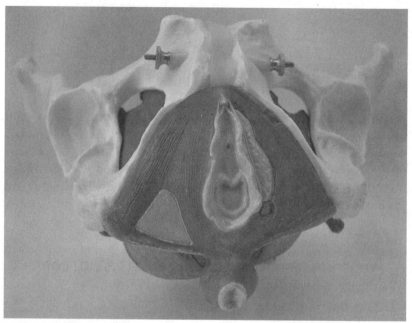

Model of the female pelvic floor muscles, with the woman lying on her back, showing the four structures that pass through the pelvic floor. Top to bottom: clitoris, urethra, vagina, rectum.

Can you tell by looking at this view that the pelvic floor is actually a *group* of muscles and not just one muscle? There are two layers, and many individual muscles, that make up the pelvic floor muscle group. When you give birth, these muscles stretch and stretch to allow the baby's head to pass through the vaginal opening. Think of a camera lens as it opens to achieve a larger aperture. This is a better design than if the pelvic floor was just one large, continuous muscle with minimal flexibility.

It is unnecessary to learn all the individual names of the pelvic floor group muscles, because they all work together. There is only one nerve that innervates all of the pelvic floor muscles (the *pudendal* nerve), so it is an all-or-none type of contraction. You cannot contract the muscles individually. This is an important concept to realize in the training process, because you can visualize squeezing just one part of the pelvic floor, and the whole thing will contract. An example of this would be squeezing as if you were trying to hold back gas, and the section around your urethra will contract as well.

We now show you four at-home ways to gain confidence that you have found your pelvic floor muscles. We will progress from less invasive to more invasive.

The "Stop Test"

Go to your toilet and urinate. In the middle of urinating, see if you can stop your urine from flowing. Can you stop your urine flow completely for a second or two? If you can, then you have found your pelvic floor muscles!

If you were not able to stop your urine flow completely for a few seconds, then your muscles are weaker and/or more uncoordinated than they should be. See if you can just slow down your stream to make it weaker or slower. Can you do this? If you can, then again, you have found your pelvic floor muscles. You must remember what this feels like, so try it again right after you are finished urinating, while you are still sitting on the toilet. Can you do the same squeeze even without urinating? The reason you will need to remember how this feels is because you will need to repeat this same squeeze or contraction when performing your home exercise program in the next chapter.

AN IMPORTANT WORD OF CAUTION: The "Stop Test" is just a test to help you locate your pelvic floor muscles. This is *not* the correct time to actually *do* your pelvic floor exercises, as part of your home treatment plan. Your ability to urinate is a delicate reflex, and you don't want to interfere with it. It doesn't feel natural to stop your urine, does it? Surely, you feel the pressure build up in your bladder. It is not advisable to stop your urination once you have begun, because this can lead to dysfunctional voiding. It is safe to repeat this test once a month to see if you are better able to stop your urine flow, but not more often. However, right *after* you urinate is a perfectly OK time to do the home exercises that you will learn soon.

The Stop Test is not so easy, and not everyone with incontinence can do it. If you weren't able to do it successfully, don't despair: There are other ways to find your pelvic floor muscles.

Hold Back Gas or a Bowel Movement

Look at the image on the previous page again. Can you see the thick, round ring of muscles circling the rectum? This part of your pelvic floor muscles gives you control over your rectal opening, allowing gas and bowel movements to pass through or stay inside.

Do you remember learning that contracting or squeezing any part of the pelvic floor will make all other pelvic floor muscles contract as well? Let's use this to our advantage. Can you hold back gas when you are in a social situation? Test this the next time you feel gas about to escape. If you can hold the gas in, you have just contracted your pelvic floor muscles.

If you can't hold back your gas, do not worry. Many incontinent women are unable to do so, and unfortunately this results in further embarrassment. As an added bonus, this odorous problem will automatically improve as you begin training your muscles to get stronger.

Try the same thing with your next bowel movement. Can you delay it for five or ten minutes? A person should have at least that much control over the feces, or he or she risks a different kind of accident called *fecal incontinence*. The control required to hold back gas and/or a bowel movement takes strong endurance and good tone of your pelvic floor muscles, and these are goals in our rehabilitative plan for you. What if you can't successfully hold back gas or bowel movements? Then let's go on to another method to find these uncooperative muscles!

Sit on a Rolled Towel

Are you sitting as you read this book? If you are sitting up straight, then you are sitting right on your pelvic floor muscles right now. They connect to your "sit bones" and are right under your skin. These bones are the ones that get sore when you sit on an unpadded bleacher while watching a sporting event.

Get a hand towel and roll it up so it is about six to eight inches long. Place this rolled-up towel on a hard chair (not on a soft, cushy couch), parallel to your thighs, so that the towel roll touches both your pubic bone (in the front) and your tailbone (in the back). This towel roll should make it easier for you to feel your pelvic floor contractions, because it gives you better surface contact with them.

Now squeeze as if you were to stop your urine flow, hold back gas or a bowel movement, or clamp your vaginal opening closed. Squeeze around the towel. Try to grab it with your muscles. Be patient and give this a few minutes before throwing in the towel. Your pelvic floor muscles are not accustomed to being used this way.

What do you feel as you squeeze the towel roll with your pelvic floor muscles? Do you feel a slight movement around the towel? If so, this is your pelvic floor working! As the pelvic floor contracts, it lifts up and off the towel in the direction of your head. The towel gives you added contact pressure and that, too, is a form of biofeedback that will help you find these hidden muscles.

Still no luck? Read on.

Vaginal Palpation

OK; now it is time to get a little personal. Just like a physical therapist or physician would want to feel your pelvic floor muscle working, so must you if the other three methods didn't work for you.

Wash your hands. Wear medical-grade examination gloves if you feel more comfortable. Lie on your back, on your bed, with your knees up and spread open in the position you are in when you have a pap smear. Ideally, you should prop up your knees so you don't have to hold them up with muscle power. Resting even one knee against a wall helps relax the leg muscles so you can focus on finding your pelvic floor.

Now take your right thumb (or left thumb if you are left-handed) and insert it into your vagina all the way. With the pad of your thumb facing downward, gently push down toward your rectum until your thumb seems to stop. You are now almost touching your pelvic floor muscles. The only thing between your muscles and your thumb is the wall of your vagina. Do not move your thumb, but keep it very still so you can concentrate on feeling your pelvic floor muscles.

Do you feel anything happening under your thumb pad? Do you feel a little movement? You may feel a weak flicker of the muscles. Do you feel your thumb lift up a little when you squeeze around it? If you do, these are your pelvic floor muscles working. Remember, do not wiggle your thumb around inside your vagina. You and your thumb must be very still to try to get a true feel of these weak muscles. If you feel anything moving, try to make that movement stronger. Try squeezing harder around your thumb. Do you feel it?

If you have *not* felt this muscle contract with any of the four at-home methods presented here, keep practicing until you do. You will not be able to progress to doing your home exercise plan without first finding these muscles. Perhaps you will need to consult with a medical professional, such as a physical therapist specializing in incontinence, who can perform SEMG biofeedback with you.

To find a local physical therapist who specializes in Women's Health or incontinence, consult your local phone book, or go to the Women's Health Section of the American Physical Therapy Association website (http://www.womenshealthapta.org/find-a-physical-therapist/index.cfm). Simply enter your zip code and you will be given the names of physical therapists in your geographic area who have the specialized training you need to help you overcome your urinary incontinence and other bladder issues. This book will be a great tool you can use to work with your physical therapist.

INSTRUCTIONS FOR FINDING YOUR PELVIC FLOOR
Try each and every cue presented in this chapter,
to find the one that works best for you:

1. When you are urinating, try to stop your stream.
2. Try to hold back gas or a bowel movement.
3. Sit on a rolled-up towel and try to squeeze around it.
4. Clamp your vagina closed, around your thumb.

We hope that one of the four methods we described did help you correctly locate your pelvic floor muscles. Now that you know how to find your pelvic floor muscles, you likely have many questions: How many exercises should you be doing? How long should you be holding the squeeze? What positions should you be doing them in?

You will receive the answers to these questions in the next chapter, because now you are ready to receive a physical therapy home treatment plan to correctly and successfully improve the strength, the endurance, the coordination, and the tone of these hidden muscles!

> "Learning is not attained by chance, it must be sought for with ardor
> and attended to with diligence."
> —Abigail Adams

3 Your Treatment Plan to End Stress Urinary Incontinence

"READY TO TAKE ACTION": REVISIT ERICA AND TERRY

*E*rica wants to dance again! She is tired of standing in the corner tapping her toes. "Tapping her toes" has become the metaphor for her life these days. She doesn't want to hesitate anymore when friends invite her on a hike, or when her husband leads her out to the dance floor at a wedding. She wants to be herself again. Standing on the sidelines as an observer is NOT who she is, but it IS who she has become.

Terry is sick of her constant focus on how to spruce up yet another dark suit. After years in the fashion business, she has accepted that black is the only color that truly hides her stains. She wants to stop lugging bulky tote bags filled with pads and spare panties . . . and get back to carrying trendy handbags. The final blow to her fragile ego came when a coworker laughed aloud while reading that Japan's growing incontinence market boasted the first-ever adult diaper fashion show. Snatching the magazine from her coworker's hands, Terry went on to read and found out that it was true!

> The adult diaper market in Japan is growing (Reuters News Service, 2007). On September 25, 2008, Japanese manufacturers of adult diapers conducted the world's first all-diaper fashion show, dramatizing through it many informative dramatic scenarios, which addressed various issues relevant to older people in diapers. "It was great to see so many types of diapers all in one showing," said Aya Habuka, 26. "I learned a lot. This is the first time that diapers are being considered as fashion." (Fox News, 2008)

Sick at heart with this news, Terry vowed this was one fashion trend she was determined to skip. Both Erica and Terry just want to feel normal again, and they are desperate to find the key to their bathroom miseries. Terry is ready *to act, and she speaks to her gynecologist at her next visit. Her doctor refers her to a urologist. Erica simply consults her family doctor. All three physicians recommend the noninvasive physical therapy approach as the first treatment to end their incontinence. The physicians know it works, because they have witnessed immense success with physical therapy in their prior patients.*

After a couple of physical therapy sessions, Erica realizes this approach is way more than "just Kegel exercises," which she also learns are actually quite different from the ones she has been doing haphazardly for years. She follows her home program religiously, and soon she can dance and jump without leaking.

Terry learns how to correctly find her pelvic floor muscles for the first time, thanks to the SEMG biofeedback. She no longer does a bridging exercise, substituting "wrong" muscles for her pelvic floor muscles. She uses vaginal weights at home to build up her endurance.

Each lady's physical therapist gives her a thorough list of home exercises to improve the strength, endurance, function, and coordination of their pelvic floor muscles—and each patient is conscientious in doing those exercises.

After a mere ten physical therapy sessions for Erica, and twelve weekly sessions for Terry, both women are dry and no longer using pads. Erica feels her life is no longer ruled by this annoying, hidden problem. Terry feels like a new woman and is thrilled to be pad-free!

This chapter is the heart of the book for those of you suffering from stress urinary incontinence. The plan we present in the following pages is the key to getting your life back. However, we want to begin with some solid advice: Take it slow. This chapter is long. It is bursting with wonderful exercise plans to get your pelvic floor fit. This plan is about learning the exercises correctly the first time. It is not a race to the finish line but rather a process that, if executed properly, is foolproof. Think quality, not speed. You must be patient with the program and with yourself.

If, like Erica and Terry, you were in a formal physical therapy program, the information you will receive in this chapter would have been doled out to you in small doses, weekly, over a period of about two months. We recommend the same approach to your home program. Follow the set schedule of exercises, and embrace the training you are doing during each phase. Learn and master it, before you go on. **Take your time**.

You may decide to read through the entire chapter and then go back and work section by section. You may wish to go week by week, matching your reading to your workout schedule. Either way is fine. This is a "working" chapter. Ideally, it should take you eight to sixteen weeks to get through the program in this chapter.

You'll need a week's time to incorporate what is being prescribed for that particular week. The program is broken down into one-week segments, and you will need all seven days to learn and perform the exercise prescribed.

As you pause between sections of this chapter, each subsequent progression of your home program will make more sense, and you won't feel overloaded with too much information. The more focused and diligent you are each week, the faster your results will come. You probably have had your incontinence for years. Give yourself these eight to sixteen weeks to overcome it! Strengthening takes time and can't be rushed.

If you take the pauses we suggest, you will be better prepared, both physically and mentally, to move on to the following week's plan. The sequence of exercises is designed to build on the progress made in the previous week. You may be tempted to hurry through or skip ahead, but please don't jeopardize your success. This physical therapy home program is a proven formula to end stress urinary incontinence—just like it did for Kim and for thousands of Kathryn's patients over the past fifteen years.

By now, you have successfully used one of the methods covered in Chapter 2 to find your pelvic floor muscles. Congratulations! Now that you have identified those muscles, it's time to teach you specific exercises to progressively and comprehensively rehabilitate your pelvic floor. Our focus will be on improving your strength, endurance, coordination, function, and muscle tone. The goal is to end your stress urinary incontinence in eight to sixteen weeks. This timetable will vary, depending on the severity of your problem and the degree of weakness of your pelvic floor muscles.

Once you have conquered your stress urinary incontinence and your pelvic floor is strong, maintenance is imperative. As with any fitness regimen (or diet program), making it part of your daily life is crucial. We will show you ways to weave these exercises into your day-to-day routine to keep your pelvic floor fit and ward off any possible return of your stress incontinence.

These are the seven categories of exercises you will perform over the next eight to sixteen weeks:

1. Exercises to improve strength
2. Exercises to improve endurance
3. Exercises to improve coordination
4. Exercises to train accessory muscles
5. Advanced exercises to improve function

6.   Advanced exercises to improve tone
7.   Advanced exercises that add resistance

Remember that the pelvic floor is a group of skeletal muscles. All skeletal muscles should possess strength, endurance, coordination, function, and good tone, and your pelvic floor muscles are no exception. As you can plainly see, the treatment plan to cure your stress urinary incontinence is much more that "just Kegel exercises."

Still, we must give Dr. Kegel credit for being the first to realize that exercising the pelvic floor muscles would alleviate stress urinary incontinence. The modern approach to muscle rehabilitation has been further developed over time, and you are about to learn the most comprehensive physical therapy home program available to end your stress urinary incontinence.

Throughout this chapter, we meticulously describe each exercise, making it crystal clear how to do each one correctly and avoid common errors. At the end of the chapter we provide a handout for your home program, a week-by-week summary of this chapter. Please photocopy this and keep it nearby as a handy reminder. Put it where you will notice it every day, such as on your refrigerator or on the mirror in your bathroom. Follow it conscientiously, and you will end your stress incontinence forever!

During Week 1 through Week 3, you will be doing a combination of two types of exercise. One will build strength, and the other will build endurance. Although each exercise is unique, they both will be performed in the same body position throughout each seven-day period. These exercises can be performed one after the other, or at different times during the day, as long as all required sets are completed. As you progress from week to week, the body positions will advance from lying down, to sitting, and finally to standing. These exercises will result in improved strength and endurance of your pelvic floor.

EXERCISES TO IMPROVE STRENGTH: WEEKS 1 THROUGH 3

Let's get underway with your exercises! Choose the method that worked best for you in Chapter 2 to locate and contract your pelvic floor muscles. To review, they are:

■   Squeeze as if to stop your urine flow.
■   Squeeze as if to hold in gas or a bowel movement.

- Squeeze while sitting on a rolled towel.
- Squeeze around your vagina, while palpating with your thumb inserted vaginally.

Use whichever method you prefer, but be sure you have confidently located and contracted your pelvic floor. If you have not done this, the following home treatment plan will not succeed.

Lie on your back. You can prop up your head with pillows if that is more comfortable. Slowly contract (squeeze) your pelvic floor muscles. As you contract, the pelvic floor lifts upward, toward your head. You should not be bearing down during the squeeze. It should not feel like a push, but rather like an **upward pull**. Pushing down (called the *Valsalva Maneuver*) is a very common mistake that women often make when they (falsely) believe they are doing their Kegels. Lying down is the easiest way to start, because your pelvic floor doesn't have to fight gravity in this position.

If you were doing this exercise while connected to a surface electromyographic (SEMG) biofeedback machine, it would look like the computer screen pictured below. Imagine the line moving along

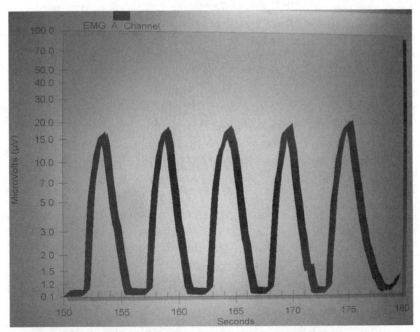

Computerized SEMG biofeedback graphs showing five quick (two-second) contractions for strength training.

with your exercises, just as an EKG line moves with every heartbeat. These visual images are vital throughout your home program. Keep them in your mind's eye as you squeeze and release your pelvic floor. As Dr. Kegel taught us, the eye-to-muscle connection is critical to your success. Try to envision the movement of the black line as you do this two-second strengthening exercise, **while looking** at the SEMG biofeedback graph on the previous page.

Were you able to imagine the black line climb higher as you squeezed your pelvic floor harder? Could you follow the line downward as you relaxed the pelvic floor? Remember this visual image, because you will use it while you exercise by keeping it in your memory as you contract your pelvic floor muscles.

You will perform **ten** quick, two-second contractions **three times a day**. Please continue doing your pelvic floor exercises in the reclined position for **one week**.

COMMON MISTAKE

Do not try to substitute other muscles in this exercise. Strive to keep your belly, your buttocks, and your inner thighs relaxed. Contract your pelvic floor muscle **only**. These other, stronger muscles would love to take over for your weaker pelvic floor. This is another good reason to begin these exercises while lying on your back, when you are more relaxed.

After this first week, we need to make the work harder for your pelvic floor muscles, just as a weight lifter uses heavier weights to get stronger. We do this by advancing your exercises into the **sitting** position in **Week 2**. This is your next progression. You do not have to do these exercises lying on your back anymore.

Sit on a hard chair rather than a cushy couch. As you contract, you may feel the pelvic floor lift upward, toward your head, like it did while you were on your back, but now you will also feel it lift off the chair. You will stay in contact with the chair, but internally you will begin to feel your pelvic floor muscles elevate above your sit bones. Sometimes this takes a few days of exercising to feel. The chair is supporting your pelvic floor muscles from underneath, so your muscles don't have to fight gravity alone—the chair helps!

In **Week 3** you will begin doing this same exercise while **standing**. By changing your positions from easier to more difficult ones, you will add more gravity and thus more resistance to your pelvic floor muscles. You do not have to do the previous exercises while sitting or lying on your back anymore.

Your pelvic floor fights the most amount of gravity in the standing position. Without the chair to support the muscles from underneath, the muscles tend to sag, or hang in the shape of a hammock. When you are standing, your pelvic floor must work extra hard to hold itself up, support all your organs, and be strong enough to keep you dry. This is why you probably have the most leakage while standing, walking, and running, because these activities further tax your pelvic floor muscles. However, this is how you build strength—by challenging your muscles to do more and more, week by week.

How long will it take before you are completely dry and no longer leaking urine when you cough or sneeze? In our own experience (and considering Kathryn has treated thousands of patients), it will be eight to sixteen weeks before you are dry and out of pads. However, you should begin to notice improvement in just a couple of weeks.

Three factors influence this time frame:

1. How bad your leakage problem was at the start of this program.
2. How active your lifestyle is; for example, it will take longer to stay dry while playing an entire tennis match than in the few seconds it takes to stand up from a chair.
3. How old you are. Naturally, all skeletal muscles get weaker as we age, but even seniors can definitely increase their pelvic floor strength over the threshold into dryness.

You will continue doing these standing quick contractions until you are dry or nearly dry: Perform ten repetitions, in three sessions per day. Later in this chapter, we show you ways to interlace pelvic floor exercises into your life, ultimately replacing the need to do these formal exercises while standing.

Be diligent with your exercises, and you will be rewarded with diminishing leakage! In a few short weeks, you will experience fewer, and smaller, leaks and you will need to wear fewer pads. Treat yourself to a lunch out with a girlfriend, or buy a new pair of shoes with the money you'll save on pads. Relish your sweet success!

As you learned earlier, your pelvic floor muscles need more than just strengthening. They need far better endurance to give you the control you desire. You will learn these endurance exercises next.

You will perform your strengthening and your endurance exercises in the same session.

NOTE: You will be performing two different exercises together. The "Quick" and the "Endurance" exercises are done in tandem, in the same session, three times a day, with ten repetitions each. Do the exercises one week in each of the three positions: (a) on your back, then (b) sitting, then (c) standing.

EXERCISES TO IMPROVE ENDURANCE: WEEKS 1 THROUGH 3

There are two types of muscle cells (or muscle fibers) in every skeletal muscle, called *Type I* and *Type II*. Type I muscle fibers move relatively quickly, whereas Type II muscle fibers move a bit more slowly. Perhaps you go to the gym to build up your upper leg strength by lifting weights thirty times, as you bend and straighten your knees. Pumping weights increases the strength in the Type I, fast-twitching muscle fibers in your quadriceps.

Because your pelvic floor muscles are skeletal muscles, they contain both Type I and Type II muscle fibers, and both types of exercise are needed to strengthen them thoroughly. Seventy percent of the muscle fibers in the pelvic floor are Type II, the slow-twitching, endurance-related variety. This makes sense, because the pelvic floor works all day long to hold up your organs. It also works all day long when trying to keep your urethra closed so that urine doesn't leak out while you are standing and walking. Conversely, you may sneeze only once a day, and that is when your Type I strength fibers are called into action.

It is very common for women to perform only the short, quick contractions that you learned in the preceding section when performing Kegel exercises. In essence, they are only exercising thirty percent of the cells in their pelvic floor muscles. This is not nearly good enough! Let's improve your holding power by learning some important endurance exercises.

Lie on your back, because this is the easiest position in which to start, with minimal gravitational influence. You can prop your head with pillows if you are more comfortable that way. Contract

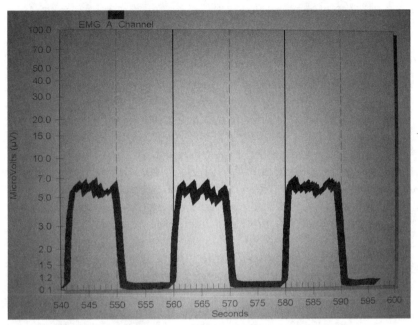

Computerized SEMG biofeedback graphs showing three long (ten-second) contractions for endurance training.

your pelvic floor and **hold** the contraction for a count of ten, before releasing and resting for another count of ten.

If you were doing this exercise while connected to an SEMG biofeedback machine, it would look like the shape above. Imagine the line moving along with your exercises, just like an EKG line moves. Can you imagine holding the contraction for ten seconds as the line goes up and stays up? Then can you see that as you let go of your muscles, the line drops back down to your baseline? Rest for ten seconds before trying the exercise again.

Try doing an endurance contraction while lying on your back, looking at the figure above and breathing normally. The spike goes up and then holds steady for a count of ten before it releases down again, as you rest for ten seconds. Can you do it? If you are unable to hold the contraction for a full ten seconds, hold it as long as you can. In a few days you should be able to make it to ten seconds.

Do not hold your breath while doing these endurance exercises. Most people have the tendency to hold their breath, strain, and push down (the *Valsalva Maneuver* we discussed earlier) when doing this ten-second contraction. You don't want to create intra-abdominal pressure by pushing down on the pelvic floor at the same time you are trying to elevate it by contracting it upward.

Counting aloud is helpful to make sure you are breathing during your exercises. Use a clock with a second hand the first few times so you can judge how fast you count, in case you are a speed demon who needs to count to twenty in order to pace out ten seconds.

As you did with the image on page 45, look at the computerized graph depicted on page 49 and memorize its basic form to help you perform these exercises. Keeping this image in your mind's eye will help you during the endurance phase of your home program. The ten seconds of rest between contractions is important to give your weak muscles time to recover before the next contraction. Strive to make each contraction as strong as the previous squeeze.

You will do these endurance contractions along with the strengthening exercises you learned in the preceding section. Both exercises are performed on your back for the first week: ten repetitions each, three sessions per day.

Again, **do not** substitute with other muscles. Strive to keep your belly, buttocks, and inner thighs relaxed. These ten-second exercises are more difficult, and you will realize that you need to focus. Please don't overdo it by squeezing harder than your pelvic floor muscles alone can handle. Overachieving is when other muscles jump in and try to substitute for your pelvic floor. In the case of pelvic floor endurance exercises, less is more.

COMMON MISTAKE

Do not hold your breath. Solve this by counting **out loud** for ten seconds as you hold the contraction. When you talk, you exhale, and thus you can't be holding your breath at the same time. Counting to yourself won't work.

Just as we did with the quick strengthening exercises you learned in the preceding section, you will change your position to **sitting** in **Week 2**, and to **standing** in **Week 3**, increasingly adding more gravity and resistance. Expect your endurance to improve along the way.

The figure opposite depicts how your endurance contractions would look on an SEMG biofeedback machine by the time you reach Week 3. See how much higher the spikes in the graphs are now? That's because your hard efforts with your home program are paying off!

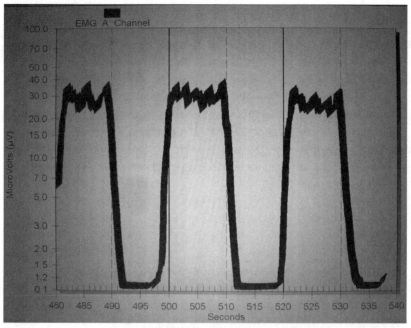

Computerized SEMG biofeedback graph.
Three long (ten-second) contractions, showing much better endurance.

Keep doing these exercises three times per day in the standing position, and you will feel the endurance in your pelvic floor muscles getting better and better. You do not have to do this endurance exercise while sitting or lying on your back anymore.

You should continue performing your ten-second endurance contractions while standing until you no longer leak urine. At that point, you will be successfully using your pelvic floor muscles throughout the day, which will be enough to maintain your endurance.

We now provide a summary of the home exercise instructions you have learned thus far, because they are done concurrently. Happy exercising!

WEEK 1

**YOUR INSTRUCTIONS FOR THE QUICK AND
ENDURANCE EXERCISES**
Position: Lying on Your Back

1. **Quick Exercise**: Squeeze your pelvic floor muscles and hold them for two seconds. Let go for two seconds, allowing your muscles to fully relax. Repeat this ten times. Perform three sessions like this per day while lying on your back. Do not use other muscles, just your pelvic floor.
2. **Endurance Exercise**: Squeeze your pelvic floor muscles and hold them for ten seconds. Let go for ten seconds, allowing your muscles to fully relax. Repeat this ten times. Perform three sessions like this per day while lying on your back. Do not hold your breath or bear down. Count out loud for ten seconds to keep breathing.

WEEK 2

YOUR INSTRUCTIONS FOR THE QUICK AND ENDURANCE EXERCISES
Position: Sitting

1. **Quick Exercise**: Squeeze your pelvic floor muscles and hold them for two seconds. Let go for two seconds, allowing your muscles to fully relax. Repeat this ten times. Perform three sessions like this per day while sitting. Do not use other muscles, just your pelvic floor.
2. **Endurance Exercise**: Squeeze your pelvic floor muscles and hold them for ten seconds. Let go for ten seconds, allowing your muscles to fully relax. Repeat this ten times. Perform three sessions like this per day while sitting. Do not hold your breath or bear down. Count out loud for ten seconds to keep breathing.

WEEK 3 AND CONTINUING UNTIL DRY

YOUR INSTRUCTIONS FOR THE QUICK AND ENDURANCE EXERCISES
Position: Standing

1. **Quick Exercise**: Squeeze your pelvic floor muscles and hold them for two seconds. Let go for two seconds, allowing your

muscles to fully relax. Repeat this ten times. Perform three sessions like this per day while standing. Do not use other muscles, just your pelvic floor.

2. **Endurance Exercise**: Squeeze your pelvic floor muscles and hold them for ten seconds. Let go for ten seconds, allowing your muscles to fully relax. Repeat this ten times. Perform three sessions like this per day while standing. Do not hold your breath or bear down. Count out loud for ten seconds to keep breathing.

> NOTE: You will continue to do your quick and endurance exercises while STANDING (three times per day as above), until you are completely DRY! Then more advanced exercises will maintain your continence.

EXERCISES TO TRAIN ACCESSORY MUSCLES: WEEK 4

Once you have been exercising your pelvic floor muscles for about three to four weeks (Week 1 on your back, Week 2 while sitting, and Week 3 while standing), you are ready to progress your exercises even further.

> NOTE: If you also have urge urinary incontinence (or urinary urgency, frequency, or nocturia), you may proceed to Chapters 4 and 5 to begin the process of retraining your bladder. This way you can begin treating your urge incontinence as you continue treating your stress incontinence. You will be following along with Chapter 3 and Chapter 5 simultaneously.

Thus far, you have been focusing very carefully to isolate your pelvic floor muscles when you exercise. You have been aware that you should not contract the muscles of your tummy, inner thighs, or buttocks. This is prudent in the early phases of rehabilitation of the pelvic floor, to ensure that these stronger muscles do not take over for your weaker pelvic floor muscles. You first had to learn to *isolate* the pelvic floor!

However, the pelvic floor does not function independently in your body. It coordinates with other muscles. There are three other muscles that serve as accessories to the pelvic floor muscles to keep you continent: (a) the deep abdominal muscles, (b) the inner thigh muscles and (c) the buttock muscles. The pelvic floor is still the *primary* muscle to cure your incontinence, but these other muscles help, too!

In this section, we teach you how to properly contract each of these three new muscles separately, and then we will bring them all together into one exercise—combining them with the pelvic floor— making a total of *four* muscles working in tandem. This new exercise is called the *accessory muscle exercise.* Now targeted as a group, these four muscles can all be worked with only one exercise. You do not have to work them separately. This not only saves time but will also feel more natural.

How to Contract the Transversus Abdominus Muscle

The *transversus abdominus muscle* is a deep abdominal muscle that is found four layers down under the skin, wrapping around your trunk like a belt. It is *not* the outermost layer of abdominals that we all recognize as the six-pack muscle in bodybuilders—that is the rectus abdominus muscle, which is targeted by the sit-up exercise. It is also not the next two layers, where the internal and external oblique muscles are found, which are used during the diagonal sit-up motion.

The transversus abdominus muscle is huge. Take a look at the sketch of it shown opposite. Can you see that this deep muscle connects from under the breastbone all the way down to the pubic bone? Notice that the fibers run horizontally, so at the waist they keep on going until they reach the next available bone: the spine. Imagine that—an abdominal muscle that covers the entire front of your belly and wraps around your waist to your spine! This deep abdominal muscle resembles a corset or a back brace, and it acts like one, too. It functions as an armor of support to your bladder.

Let's find your transversus abdominus muscle. The Pilates exercise approach (which you will learn about in Chapter 6) targets this deep abdominal muscle along with the pelvic floor. We will borrow the most popular Pilates cue by telling you to "bring your navel to your spine." Your pelvis and back should not move. Nothing should move except your belly button in an inward direction. To use another popular Pilates mantra, "Keep breathing." You are not "sucking" in your belly by holding your breath, because you should be breathing normally.

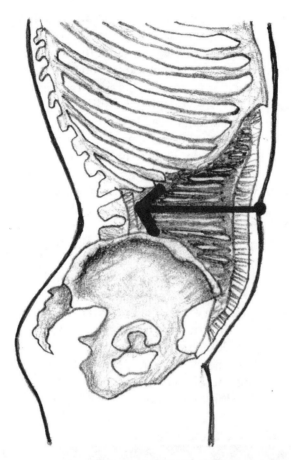

Transversus abdominus muscle attaching from the ribs, to the pubic bone, to the spine. To contract this muscle, draw your navel in toward your spine.

Another good piece of imagery to help find this deep abdominal muscle is to pretend you are zipping up a pair of jeans that are too tight. What would you do to get the zipper up? You would draw in your tummy. That's your transversus abdominus giving you a flatter tummy to allow that zipper to zip.

Try this palpation. Gently dig your index and middle fingertips into your belly—above your hip bone (called the *anterior superior iliac spine*) and below your ribs. Bring your navel in to your spine and feel the muscle harden up under your fingertips, almost trying to push your fingertips away. You can actually feel this deep abdominal muscle contract as it wraps around your waist toward your back. If you put your fingers on both sides above your hips and contract, you can really feel the sensation of a belt tightening. You may even feel it at your spine because it is contracting there as well. Remember to keep your fingers still so you can self-examine properly. The hand placement is pictured below.

Your bladder is right behind the lower portion of this transversus abdominus muscle. If you were to peel this muscle away, you'd see all your organs. This muscle supports the bladder in the front, just as the pelvic floor muscle supports the bladder from underneath. They are close cousins: Both attach to the pubic bone and the spine, and both support the bladder.

Here is a somewhat silly analogy. If your pelvic bone is like a bowl, and your organs are the fruit in the bowl, then this deep abdominal muscle acts like plastic wrap, holding and supporting all of your the organs. The pelvic floor acts like the sieve at the bottom of the fruit bowl, allowing excess water to drain off the fruit.

Both the pelvic floor and the transversus abdominus muscles are called *core muscles*. Both are deep postural supportive muscles, and neither one moves the skeleton to produce motion. Yet the transversus abdominus muscle has many important roles that athletes, dancers, and celebrities have known about for years.

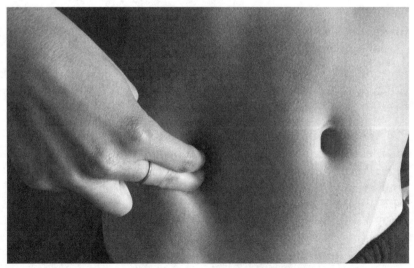

Hand placement to find the transversus abdominus muscle.

First, the transversus abdominus is the muscle that gives you a flatter tummy. (Now that we have your attention!) A sit-up won't give you a flat stomach. That's right: Doing a sit-up contracts the "six-pack" muscle (*rectus abdominus*), which is the narrow band of muscle running vertically, from your breastbone (or *sternum*) to pubic bone. It doesn't even lie around your entire tummy or at your waist in order to make it flat. The transversus abdominus muscle does!

Second, a strong transversus abdominus muscle allows you to have better posture, giving you the strength to stand up straight and tall. You know how good dancers look. Their tall elegant posture is a graceful side effect of years of strengthening this deep abdominal muscle.

Third, this deep muscle improves our balance. Because it wraps around our waist it serves to help keep our hips level when we walk, greatly aiding our balance. The shuffling gait of an elder is usually due, at least in part, to weakness in this muscle and the resultant inability to momentarily stand on one foot to take each step.

TRY THIS BALANCE TEST

Stand in your usual and most comfortable posture: stomach relaxed, shoulders at ease. Now raise your right knee toward the ceiling, causing you to balance on your left leg. How long can you hold the pose? Are you wavering? Now try it again, but before you lift your leg, bring your navel in to your spine and engage your transversus abdominus. Were you able to keep balanced longer with your muscular corset cinched tight? Did you feel steadier? We'll bet you did! This is the beauty of the transversus abdominus muscle.

Fourth, and this is the reason *we* are so interested in the transversus abdominal muscle, is that it acts to support the bladder in the front. Indeed, it does a wonderful job of supporting the bladder, which is right behind it in the lower portion of this muscle, above the pubic bone. If this muscle is strong, it will help keep the pressure of coughing, sneezing, and lifting away from the bladder. This will greatly reduce the leakage of stress urinary incontinence. We cover these and many more functional activities in the next section. For now, suffice it to say that this deep, hidden muscle is the second most important muscle in keeping you dry—following the pelvic floor, of course!

The final two muscles you need to brush up on in order to control your stress incontinence, the inner thighs and the buttocks, are (thankfully) more straightforward than the pelvic floor or the transversus abdominus muscles. Hooray!

How to Contract the Inner Thighs

The inner thighs contain a large group of muscles called the *hip adductors*. These muscles bring your legs together. In this exercise you will be using them isometrically; this means you will learn how to strengthen them without actually moving your hips or your legs. You do this by simply squeezing your heels together with your feet in a "V" position, heels touching but toes apart.

Anatomists have discovered that there is a small slip or portion of the adductor muscles that wraps around the urethra, aiding with continence.

How to Contract the Buttocks

The word *buttocks* (from which the word *butt* originates) was made familiar in the movie "Forrest Gump." It is also known as the derriere, rump, bottom, tush, cheeks, ass, fanny, and gluteals, as well as its medical name, the *gluteus maximus muscle*. If you are lying on your back and you squeeze your buttocks together, your pelvis should automatically rise up without any effort from your back, merely because the buttocks are going from soft to hard, elevating the pelvis.

OK, now let's put **all four** muscles together in order to train your pelvic floor in coordination with the three **accessory muscles**.

WEEK 4 AND CONTINUING BEYOND

YOUR INSTRUCTIONS TO TRAIN THE PELVIC FLOOR PLUS ACCESSORY MUSCLES
Position: Lying on Your Back

Lie on your back with a pillow under your knees and your heels touching, toes apart. You may elevate your head with pillows or sit up in bed, if you wish.

- **First muscle:** Contract your **pelvic floor** muscle and **hold it.**
- **Add the second muscle**: Contract your **transversus abdominus** muscle by bringing your navel to your spine. This is like trying to zip up a pair of jeans that are too tight. **Add this contraction to the pelvic floor and hold both muscles.**
- **Add the third muscle**: **Squeeze your heels** together. Add this muscle to the first two muscles and **hold all three muscles.**
- **Add the fourth muscle**: **Squeeze your buttocks** together. If you are doing this correctly, you'll feel your pelvis rise up slightly, automatically. **Hold this muscle along with the other three muscles.**
- **Hold all four muscles together, at the same time, for ten seconds.**
- **Do ten repetitions. Perform this once a day.**

Now you have learned an exercise that incorporates three additional muscles, assisting the pelvic floor in the goal of keeping you dry. When you are lying in bed or watching TV with your legs stretched out, do this exercise. It teaches you how to coordinate the pelvic floor with three other muscles. You will do this new exercise *in addition to* the quick and endurance contractions that you are currently doing in the standing position (three sets of ten each, every day).

Take a week's break to incorporate this new four-in-one exercise. When you return, you will learn how to coordinate exercising your pelvic floor with your day-to-day activities.

EXERCISES TO IMPROVE FUNCTION: WEEK 5

So, now you are doing your quick two-second contractions and your ten-second endurance contractions ten times each, three times a day, in the standing position. When you are lying down, you are performing the accessory muscle exercise you just learned. But what are you doing the *rest* of the time—while you are living life, going about your daily activities?

You need more leak-defying tips. Your pelvic floor muscles were designed to participate *in* your life, not to be muscles you work out three or four times a day for a few minutes and don't think about for the rest of the day. It is imperative to introduce pelvic floor muscle exercises into your daily functional activities, and that is exactly what we do in this section.

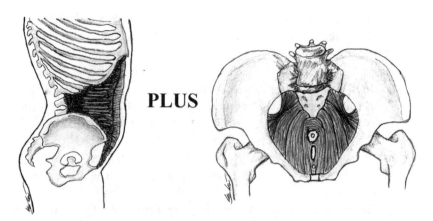

The pelvic brace (also called the *Pilates core*): transversus abdominus muscle plus the pelvic floor muscles contracting simultaneously.

In this fifth week of your home program, we add **motion** to your exercises. You will learn to coordinate two muscles (that you already know all about) with activities such as coughing, sneezing, lifting, climbing stairs, and standing up from a chair. These two muscles are the (a) pelvic floor and the (b) transverse abdominus muscles. You learned how to correctly contract the pelvic floor in Chapter 2, and in this chapter you have learned how to correctly contract the transversus abdominus.

When these two muscles are contracted together, we use the term *pelvic brace*. In a Pilates exercise program you may hear it called the *Pilates core*. These two terms are essentially synonymous. The figure above is a sketch of the pelvic brace.

Notice that both the pelvic floor and the transverse abdominus muscle connect to the pubic bone and to the spine. They are both close anatomical neighbors and core muscles. The organs are right behind your transversus abdominus and directly above your pelvic floor, so these are the deepest muscles in your pelvic region. Thus, it will feel natural to exercise them at the same time, in order to lend support to your bladder.

How to Do the Pelvic Brace

To contract these two muscles, sit on a firm chair. Squeeze your pelvic floor muscles. You should feel the pelvic floor lift up and off the chair, as these muscles move upward, toward your head. Now keep holding the pelvic floor muscles and also bring your navel in, toward your spine. This adds the transversus abdominal muscle to the pelvic floor contraction. Can you hold *both* muscles at the same time? If so, you are doing a pelvic brace, or using the Pilates core muscles.

This pelvic brace activity is not an exercise by itself; it is something you are going to add into your daily activities. This will have several important advantages.

First, it will be a way to minimize or eliminate your leakage with some of the common activities that trigger it, such as coughing and sneezing.

Second, it will add resistance to your pelvic floor and transversus abdominus muscles, further strengthening these muscles.

Third, using these muscles with daily motions you already do—such as standing up from a chair—will give you "bonus" strengthening time without devoting any additional time to your home program. You were going to stand up anyway!

Fourth, if you *do* have a busy day with no time to do your formal exercises while standing, you will not lose ground if you do the pelvic brace throughout your day during regular activities.

Fifth, once these exercises become a habitual part of your daily routine, they will actually *replace* the formal standing exercises you are currently doing. But not yet—not until you are dry! For now, you will *add* them to what you are currently doing: thirty daily quick and endurance contractions in the standing position (divided into three sessions of ten each), plus your accessory muscle exercise, while lying on your back.

Remember the pressure gradient you learned about in Chapter 2? If you can keep the pressure from getting to your bladder and pelvic floor, you will have little or no leakage with physical stress. Have you ever seen a guy ask for a punch in the gut? First he tightens up! The force of the punch is not transferred to his abdominal organs, so he feels no pain; however, if he is not ready or braced, the punch can actually damage his organs.

As the story goes, the great magician Houdini had a habit of showing off the strength of his deep abdominals by asking other men to punch him as hard as they could. One day, he got punched before he was ready—before he contracted his transversus abdominus. He suffered internal bleeding and died during his next performance from this blow to his abdominal area.

The analogy we are providing here is that during every cough, every sneeze, and every jump, you apply pressure to your abdominal organs (including your bladder), and these activities act like a punch; however, if you successfully tighten your trans-versus abdominus and pelvic floor *before*, *during*, and *slightly after* these activities, you will protect your bladder from getting all this extra pressure. The pelvic floor does its part by tightening around your urethra, thereby keeping the urine where it belongs—in your bladder—even during heavy activities.

The deep abdominals protect the bladder in front. The pelvic floor protects the bladder from underneath. Acting as a unit, the pelvic brace puts your bladder into a protective muscular corner, tipping the scale so that *you* win the pressure gradient war.

In the following sections we describe some of the most common activities that provoke stress urinary incontinence. By adding the pelvic brace to these common daily activities, you will minimize your leakage tremendously!

Coughing

Coughing is one of the most common daily activities causing uri-nary leakage. If you are sick—with the flu, for example—the leak-age with coughing intensifies.

TRY THIS COUGHING TEST

Sit on a firm chair and cough forcefully **without** doing the pelvic brace. You probably will feel your pelvic floor muscles **bulge** downward into the seat of the chair. Do you? **Now** do the **pelvic brace**: Draw your tummy in, and squeeze your pelvic floor up. Repeat the cough. Do you feel **less bulging** of your pelvic floor down toward the chair? Good! That means you now possess the strength to counteract or resist that downward pressure on your pelvic floor from the cough!

The ability of your pelvic floor to play tug-of-war against the pressure from your cough is like putting a weight on it, like adding resistance. Every time you do a pelvic brace with coughing, it builds more strength in your pelvic floor muscle in addition to preventing leakage—a double whammy benefit!

You usually do not have much time or much warning before a cough comes on. But you normally *do* have enough time to get your hand (or your elbow) to your mouth, right? You'll need to take advantage of this time and contract the two muscles of the pelvic brace as your hand is traveling toward your mouth. This takes a bit of coordination. Try it. Can you contract your pelvic floor and your transversus abdominus muscles, while your hand is moving toward your mouth? Good.

Now add the cough. *Hold* the pelvic brace (i.e., the pelvic floor and transversus abdominus muscles) slightly before, during, and slightly after your cough while your hand is moving toward your mouth. Think of this as an endurance contraction, because you don't know whether you are going to cough once or six times in a row. It is important to keep holding the pelvic brace as long as you are still coughing. You wouldn't want to stay dry for the first two coughs and then leak on the third cough!

Once your cough is over and your arm goes down, you can also relax your pelvic brace. Think of your hand as the lever that turns your pelvic brace *on* before the cough and turns the brace *off* after the cough is finished.

Sneezing

All the same principles apply with sneezing as with coughing, and the technique is identical. Thinking of your arm as the lever, contract the two muscles of the pelvic brace before, during, and a little after your sneeze. Envision your hand or elbow traveling to and from your mouth as a lever turning these muscles on and then off. How many times in a row do you sneeze? For most people, it is more than once. Don't let go of your pelvic brace before your second sneeze, or you will stay dry during the first sneeze but leak on the second sneeze. Do the pelvic brace before, during, and after laughing and blowing your nose, too. All the same principles apply.

Standing Up from a Chair

Whereas you may not cough or sneeze in an entire day, you will stand up thirty to sixty times in a day. You'll stand up from your bed, toilet, kitchen chair, living room couch, desk chair, and car. If you successfully learn to do the pelvic brace before standing up, your leakage will decrease substantially.

Let's first learn some important body mechanics to lessen the pressure on your bladder. The *way* you stand up can be causing a lot of your leakage. Here is the proper way to stand up from a chair:

- Slide forward to the edge of your chair.
- Put your feet back and under you, so that your heels are almost ready to pop up off the floor. Your feet should be hip-width apart.
- Do the pelvic brace: Draw your navel in toward your spine, and squeeze your pelvic floor.
- Use the armrests if you have them. *Hold* the pelvic brace, and stand up.

This technique should be much easier than straining to get up when your body weight is far back, deep in the chair. The legs have a much better mechanical advantage with the method we just described. By rising from a sitting position in this way, you actually create less pressure on your bladder and pelvic floor (and on your back). What pressure still remains is offset by your pelvic brace, and leakage will be prevented or minimized.

The hardest thing about doing the pelvic brace is not learning it, but *remembering* it. The good news is that if you forget to do the brace when you stand up and you get a squirt of urine leakage, this will only help you better remember next time. It's called *negative reinforcement* and is a very good way to learn something new.

The eventual goal is not having to even *think* about sliding forward and doing the pelvic brace while standing up, because it has become automatic—just like it's automatic to cover your mouth when you cough. Practice this as many times as you remember, and soon it will become your new and improved way of standing up from a chair.

Squatting

Starting from the standing position, hold the pelvic brace and do a small mini-squat. This helps you disassociate your pelvic brace from your leg joints. See, it is possible to keep hold of your pelvic brace while you move your hips, knees, and ankles. Do this while you squat to empty the dishwasher, take clothes out of the dryer, or reach into a low shelf.

Lifting

Once you have mastered squatting, try lifting. Again, it is very important to use proper body mechanics while lifting, in order to minimize the pressure on your bladder, on your pelvic floor, and on your back. The following steps list the proper way to lift something from the floor:

- Get as close to the object as you can. If possible, place your feet alongside the object. Placing your feet in a diagonal stance will also help, because it gives more room for your knees to bend without bumping into the item you are lifting. Bend with your knees, not with your back, to reach the object. This is the squat you just learned.
- As you touch the object you are about to lift, contract your pelvic brace firmly. Draw your navel in toward your spine and squeeze to elevate your pelvic floor.
- **Hold** the pelvic brace and **lift** the object. **Keep** the pelvic brace as you carry the object to wherever you are taking it.

As you lift your laundry basket with this technique, you will prevent leakage while protecting your bladder (and your back). If you are lifting a casserole dish from a table or a pot of spaghetti from the stove, you should use the same technique, even though no squatting is involved. Try to think about all the common things you lift each day and try to do it this way. It may feel a bit different at first, but the payoff—less leakage— will be well worth it!

Lunges

Lunging is an activity that really magnifies the important role the pelvic brace plays in walking. Here is another experiment for you:

- Stand and put your hands on your hips at the waist (on the *iliac crest* of your pelvis). Do *not* do the pelvic brace.
- Lift your right leg and notice what happens to your right hip. Did your right hip tip downward? Did you feel like you were beginning to lose your balance, falling to the right?
- Next, repeat the above, except *do* the pelvic brace before lifting your right leg. Draw your navel in toward your spine and squeeze to elevate your pelvic floor. Again, notice what happens to your right hip. Do your hips stay level? Do you feel more balanced?

Any female ballet dancer has an ironclad pelvic brace, or she would never be able to rise up onto one toe shoe. As we walk we need this same strength, because walking involves temporarily balancing on one leg. Have you ever noticed the way some elderly people shuffle as they walk, never really lifting their feet? This may be due to weak core muscles that prevent them from balancing on one leg long enough to lift their feet, in order to walk normally.

Do **lunging** exercises while standing:

- Contract your pelvic brace. Draw your navel in toward your spine and squeeze your pelvic floor.
- Place your hands on your hips and strive to keep your hips level. Take a small step forward with your right foot. Bend both knees.
- Bring your right foot back alongside your left foot. Repeat this lunge with your left foot. Do five repetitions on each foot, for a total of ten repetitions.
- You can relax the pelvic brace between each repetition, or—as you get stronger—you can hold it while you do all ten repetitions.
- Perform this exercise **once** a day.

You can do this as an individual exercise, or you can do it casually, for example, whenever you vacuum. Gym-goers may hold weights in their hands for added strengthening.

Stair Climbing

Once you have mastered lunging with your pelvic brace, stairs are next. The act of climbing stairs is similar to lunges but involves the added stress of lifting your entire body weight up from one step to the next. Your pelvic brace should be engaged by the time your foot lands on the first step. Now try to *hold* the brace for a full flight of steps. If there are ten steps, this may take about ten seconds, which is the same as the endurance contraction you have learned. Once you arrive at the top of the flight of stairs, you can relax your pelvic brace.

You should contract your pelvic brace when descending stairs, too. Just as with the lunge, try to keep your hips level (held that way by your pelvic brace) as you climb or descend the stairs. A bonus is that your legs will work more efficiently if they are connected to a firm core (rather than a weak and floppy midsection), and you may notice that it actually feels easier to climb stairs this way!

Sports

Once you have achieved dryness with the preceding functional activities, it is time to try adding the pelvic brace into your athletic activities. This will be much more difficult, so don't expect immediate success. Whereas not leaking when getting up from a chair may take just a few weeks to achieve, staying dry during heavy exercise and sports may take several months. This is because the pressure placed on your bladder and pelvic floor is *huge*, whenever you jump to play beach volleyball, run two miles, or do high forceful kicking during a kickboxing class. Begin by trying to hold the pelvic brace intermittently, as you lift weights at the gym. Your pelvic floor will need an ultimate amount of strength to counteract the high demand placed on it by athletic activity. If your leakage has been occurring for years, it won't resolve overnight. It will resolve eventually, though, so keep exercising your pelvic floor and you will definitely see gradual progress.

Endurance activities, such as walking on a golf course, hiking, running, skiing, or playing several sets of tennis, will present an even bigger challenge. You will need some advanced exercises to increase your coordination and tone and to add more resistance. Read on—those exercises are covered in the next three sections of this chapter.

By now you should be getting the idea. You can pretty much add the pelvic brace to *any* activity you routinely perform. Certainly you should add it to any activity that causes you leakage. Maybe you garden. Maybe you routinely make photocopies in your workplace. Couple the pelvic brace with taking your daily medications or vitamins—tasks you are unlikely to forget. For example, some women link their pelvic brace exercises to mealtimes, holding the brace while setting the table, carrying the food, and clearing the table. They don't forget to eat three times a day, so they never forget to do their pelvic brace exercises, either!

Associating the pelvic brace with tasks *you already do* increases the likelihood that you will successfully weave it into your life. As you experience fewer leaks and buy fewer pads, you will be motivated to stay compliant with blending your pelvic brace exercises into your life.

WEEK 5 AND CONTINUING BEYOND

**YOUR INSTRUCTIONS FOR THE PELVIC BRACE
TO IMPROVE FUNCTION
Position: Various**

1. **Contract the pelvic brace:** Draw your navel in toward your spine and squeeze your pelvic floor.
   Do the pelvic brace whenever you cough, sneeze, laugh, blow your nose, stand up from a chair, squat, lift, lunge, climb stairs, or do sports.
2. **Add** the pelvic brace to **any** activity that causes leakage.
3. **Add** the pelvic brace to activities you already do routinely in your life—such as meals and taking vitamins/medications.

WHEW! This was a big, important section! Take one week (or perhaps even two weeks) to incorporate all of this. Then get ready to learn some fun advanced coordination exercises!

ADVANCED EXERCISES TO IMPROVE COORDINATION: WEEK 6

Are you successfully using the pelvic brace with your daily activities as you learned in the last section (or at least much of the time)? Are you still doing the exercises from the first three sections of this chapter while standing and lying down? Are you experiencing less leakage because of all this hard work?

If you answered "yes" to all of these questions, then you are ready for some more advanced exercises. The two new exercises in this section are designed to build coordination in your pelvic floor muscles. All skeletal muscles need coordination, and the pelvic floor is no exception.

The first advanced coordination exercise is called the *combination exercise*. It combines two exercises with which you are already very familiar: an endurance contraction followed by a few quick contractions (with no rest in between). Note that this exercise is for the pelvic floor only, not the pelvic brace.

The sitting position will help you feel this advanced exercise a bit easier, because of the added contact your pelvic floor makes with the chair. Adding a towel roll will augment this sensation even further. Remember, your pelvic floor muscles are right under your skin, so they should be easy to feel while sitting on a towel roll.

WEEK 6 AND CONTINUING BEYOND

YOUR INSTRUCTIONS FOR THE "COMBINATION" COORDINATION EXERCISE
Position: Sitting

- Sit on a firm chair with a small towel roll under you, placed lengthwise behind your pubic bone and in front of your tailbone, parallel to your legs. A hand towel is an ideal size.
- Contract your pelvic floor muscles as if to do an endurance contraction, but hold the contraction for five seconds only (instead of the ten seconds you learned previously).
- Without relaxing or letting go of the pelvic floor, jump right into doing three or four quick contractions. This should take about five seconds also.
- This combination exercise should take a total of ten seconds.
- Let go of the muscle to relax it fully. Rest for ten seconds.
- Repeat this exercise five times, once a day.

The photo on the next page depicts how a SEMG biofeedback graph might look while you are doing the combination exercise. Can you imagine the line going up and holding for five seconds, and then going higher yet as you do three or four more intense, quick contractions? The entire contraction lasts ten seconds, and you must remember to relax for ten seconds before the next one.

What makes this combination exercise more difficult is that it forces a quick transition from the Type II, slow-twitching, endurance muscle fiber to the Type I, fast-twitching, strength muscle fiber. With practice, your pelvic floor will be doing the "Combo" in no time!

This combination exercise is done in *addition* to your standing exercises (the ten quick contractions and the ten endurance contractions—three times a day) and your accessory muscle exercise (on your back).

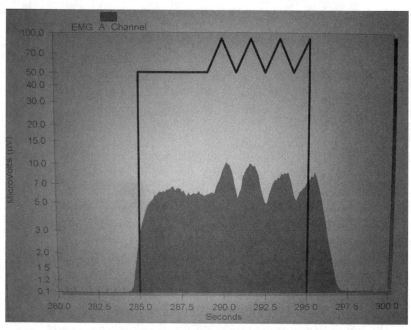

Computerized SEMG biofeedback graph showing the combination exercise for coordination training.

Here is another advanced coordination exercise for your pelvic floor, called the *stair exercise*. Please note that it does not involve climbing actual stairs.

WEEK 6 AND CONTINUING BEYOND

YOUR INSTRUCTIONS FOR THE "STAIR" COORDINATION EXERCISE
Position: Sitting

- Sit on a firm chair with a small towel roll under you, placed lengthwise behind your pubic bone and in front of your tailbone, parallel to your legs. A hand towel is an ideal size.
- Contract your pelvic floor muscles as if to do a strong endurance contraction, but hold it for five seconds only.
- Without fully letting go of the muscle, shift into doing another endurance contraction, but make this one about half effort. You

are relaxing your muscles halfway and holding them for another five seconds at a submaximal level.

■ The stair exercise should take a total of ten seconds to perform.
■ Let go of the pelvic floor to relax it fully. Rest for ten seconds.
■ Repeat this exercise for five repetitions, once a day.

The photo below shows what an SEMG biofeedback graph might look while you are doing the stair exercise. Can you imagine the line going up and holding for five seconds, then dropping half-way and holding there for another five seconds? Try to visualize this as you do your stair exercise.

What makes the stair exercise challenging is the second part, the five seconds in which you contract and hold with only half effort. Contracting a muscle in an all-or-none manner is easy for the muscle and requires little coordination; however, contracting a muscle with partial effort takes real coordination, but this is how we do our functional tasks throughout the day. Rarely do we use full effort to lift, using maximum strength. Conversely, rarely do we do nothing with our muscles. Controlled movement takes place

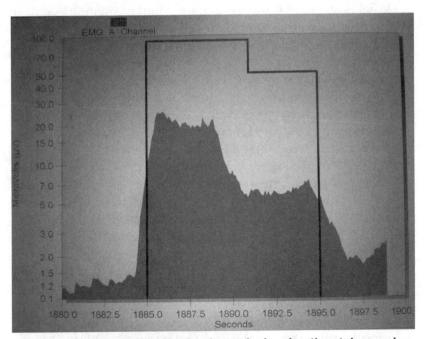

Computerized SEMG biofeedback graph showing the stair exercise for coordination training.

between these two extremes. Now your pelvic floor has learned some coordination!

Did the combination and the stair exercises remind you of the Etch-a-Sketch toy that was popular in the 1960s and 1970s? They are certainly similar, and both require advanced fine-motor muscle coordination.

By performing the combination and the stair exercises in the same session, you will have a total of ten repetitions to do while sitting (five of each). So, if you find yourself sitting and watching TV, do these exercises at commercial time!

Take a week or so to practice these two new coordination exercises while sitting. Next, we teach you how to improve the tone of your pelvic floor muscles.

ADVANCED EXERCISES TO IMPROVE TONE: WEEK 7

If you spend a lot of time on your feet, or do prolonged physical activity of any kind (i.e., that causes leakage), then you need more tone and endurance in your pelvic floor muscles.

What is *tone*? Think of tone as the amount of strength you have in your muscles when you are not even trying to contract them. It is your baseline amount of strength before contracting. Good tone and good endurance are mandatory while running, dancing, and playing sports. You may even need to get some weights.

No, we are not kidding. You can actually put weights on the pelvic floor muscle! Appropriately, they are called *vaginal weights*, and you insert them into your vagina and try to hold them in place, using your pelvic floor muscles. A weight will fall out if you are not strong enough to hold it inside your vagina. The set contains five progressively heavier weights (resembling tampons in size, with strings attached). The photo opposite shows a set of vaginal weights.

These vaginal weights are optional additions to your home program. They are an effective way to tone your pelvic floor muscles as you go about your daily chores. You don't have to just stand there as you use them. Wash your dishes. Fold your laundry. Make your bed. Do your functional exercises from the last section. Use them at home, however, *not* while out running your errands!

If you have never used tampons, you may not feel comfortable inserting these weights, but they are a great way to build tone in your pelvic floor muscles to give you added endurance with prolonged standing, running, and other sports that require lots of endurance.

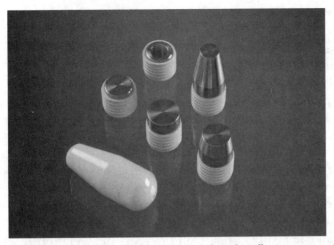

The StepFree vaginal weight system, showing five progressive weights that insert into a tampon-sized casing to increase the tone of the pelvic floor. Used with permission from SRS Medical Corporation, Redmond, Washington.

The tone that you will gain from these weights will also help you in the bedroom. Leaking while having sex is common with women who have stress incontinence, and these weights help to control that. They are also most helpful to build the tone needed to overcome nighttime bedwetting (nocturnal enuresis), yet the weights are still used during the daytime. Discount ordering information can be found in Appendix IV, page 251.

WEEK 7 AND CONTINUING BEYOND

YOUR INSTRUCTIONS TO IMPROVE TONE USING THE STEPFREE VAGINAL WEIGHT SYSTEM
Position: Various

How to progress from the lightest (first) to the heaviest (fifth) weight:

- Start with the lightest weight and screw it into the white plastic housing. Lie on your back and insert it so that it sits above your pelvic floor muscles (about two inches into your vagina). Stand up. Does the weight stay in? Does it stay in for a full minute? If it does, you may experiment with the second weight.

- If the second weight does not stay in for a full minute, then go back and use the first weight. (The first, lightest weight will most likely be the right one for you, as holding the weight in place is not always easy at first.)

Beginning with the weight you are able to hold in for one minute, stay with this same weight until you can hold it in for about fifteen minutes. Use the weights in the privacy of your home.

- Wash your dishes. Fold your laundry. Make your bed. Do some of the advanced exercises to improve coordination presented earlier in this chapter. Wearing underwear is prudent, so when a weight slips out—and it will—it won't hit the floor and roll under the couch. It is fine to reinsert the weight if it does slip out, assuming it is still clean.
- Once your initial weight can be easily held in for fifteen minutes, you can advance to the next heavier one. You can use the vaginal weights as often as you like, but usually once a day (or even less often) is fine.
- Wash the weights thoroughly with soap and water between each use. (Ordering information with discount pricing can found in Appendix IV, page 251.)

ADVANCED EXERCISES TO ADD RESISTANCE: WEEK 8

Whereas vaginal weights improve tone and endurance, there is another device on the market that will actually add resistance *directly* to your pelvic floor contractions. It is called the KegelMaster®. If you have leakage with heavy activity only, or are a serious athlete, you may opt to invest in this effective piece of equipment. This device, shown on the next page, provides varying resistance to your pelvic floor muscles for some serious strengthening.

We realize the KegelMaster® looks rather phallic. How could it not? It is inserted into your vagina, and any other shape would not suffice. As you can see in the picture, it is a hinged device with springs inside. These springs put resistance on your pelvic floor as you squeeze, thereby closing the KegelMaster®.

There are a total of *four* identical springs in the KegelMaster®, but where you place them within the unit determines how much resistance you feel. By moving the spring closer to the hinge (easier) or

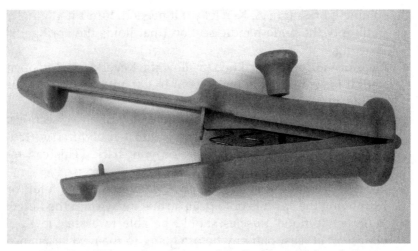

**The KegelMaster® resistive pelvic floor exercising device,
showing two (of the four) springs.**

farther from the hinge (more difficult), you can use the four springs in varying combinations to give you a total of fifteen different resistance levels.

Purchasing a KegelMaster® is optional to your home program. It comes with an instructional DVD, narrated by an medical doctor. Discount ordering information can be found in Appendix IV, page 251.

WEEK 8 AND CONTINUING BEYOND

**YOUR INSTRUCTIONS TO ADD RESISTANCE
USING THE KEGELMASTER®
Position: Lying on Your Back**

- View the ten-minute instructional KegelMaster® DVD.
- You must experiment to find which of the fifteen resistance levels is best for you. The easiest place to begin is by placing one spring on the peg closest to the hinge. Tighten the knob to close the KegelMaster®.
- Lie on your back with your knees bent and open. Position the closed KegelMaster® with the knob facing up. Use a water-

soluble lubricant (e.g., K-Y Jelly®) if needed. Insert it vaginally until only the wide handle section (that holds the springs) is showing.

■ Once inside, loosen the knob to allow the KegelMaster® to open until it fits comfortably inside you. It will not stretch out your vagina; instead, it tightens and tones.

■ Do your daily exercises as instructed in the first two sections: Ten quick (two-second) contractions and ten endurance (ten-second) contractions, while lying on your back. (This can replace a set of your standing exercises.)

■ Progress by adding additional springs (four springs total) or by moving the springs onto pegs farther away from the hinge. Your pelvic floor muscles should be able to close the KegelMaster® at least halfway before going to the next resistance level.

■ When finished exercising, pinch the KegelMaster® closed with your hands, tighten the knob, and slide it out.

■ Wash it thoroughly with soap and water between each use. You can wash and store the KegelMaster® without removing the springs. Ordering information with discount pricing is found in Appendix IV, page 251.)

■ **Do not use the KegelMaster®** with other intravaginal devices, such as tampons, diaphragms, or pessaries.
■ **Wait at least six weeks** to use it after a vaginal delivery or pelvic surgery.

BONUS EXERCISES

**TO CONTROL LEAKAGE
DURING SEXUAL INTERCOURSE**

It takes colossal pelvic floor strength and endurance to not experience leakage during sexual intercourse, when the vaginal portion of the pelvic floor is being directly impacted.

Medical literature cites the occurrence of urinary leakage during sexual activity as falling somewhere between eleven percent and sixty percent of women with stress urinary incontinence (Barber, Mullen, et al., 2005, pp. 225–232). Fortunately, studies support our own experience that physical therapy helps eradicate this problem. One controlled study reported that, after a pelvic floor exercise program, incontinence during intercourse dropped by nearly fifty percent; the overall sex life of the women in the study improved as well (Bo, Talseth, & Vinsnes, 2000).

Advanced pelvic floor exercises are needed to help you enhance endurance, tolerate resistance, and build tone to overcome leakage during sex. Both vaginal weights and the KegelMaster® provide excellent ways to prevent stress incontinence during intercourse. The Super Kegel and Glazer's Protocol are two other advanced exercises that will also help.

Super Kegel

By holding the traditional (ten-second) endurance contraction for twenty seconds instead (or longer), you can further improve your endurance. Do ten ultralong repetitions like this every day to reduce leakage during sexual intercourse. You can do this with a KegelMaster® to add even more strengthening. Maintaining a long contraction during sex, called the "hug your man" exercise, will have the added bonus of improving sexual appreciation for both partners while reducing leakage at the same time.

Glazer's Protocol

Robert Glazer, MD, has developed rehabilitation protocols for the pelvic floor. He recommends ten-second squeezes, followed by ten seconds of rest, performed sixty times (equaling twenty minutes), twice a day, to build endurance.

Realize that these bonus exercises are not exclusive to leakage during sex. They will benefit anyone and will only make your pelvic floor stronger.

Your success is rooted in your devotion. You have shown incredible perseverance to get to this point—eight (plus) weeks into your home program to end your stress urinary incontinence! You made it! It was not always so easy—but we strived to give you understandable, detailed information about the seven types of exercise to comprehensively strengthen your pelvic floor.

For your added convenience, we now provide you with a **12-week summary** of the exercises presented in this chapter, to put it all together in an easy-to-follow timeline format. If you are unsure about any of the exercises, please go back and review them in this chapter. Adjust this general timeline as your ability requires.

Please photocopy this home program and keep it in a handy spot for easy reference. Tape it on your bathroom mirror. Keep following it as your treasure map to the state of dryness!

YOUR HOME PROGRAM FOR STRESS URINARY INCONTINENCE

TWELVE-WEEK SUMMARY

Please modify this general timeline according to your ability.

■ **Week 1**
PURPOSE: To build strength and endurance

Lying on your back:

■ Squeeze your pelvic floor muscles for two seconds. Then rest for two seconds. Repeat this ten times, three sessions per day.

■ Squeeze your pelvic floor muscles and hold for ten seconds, then rest for ten seconds. Repeat this ten times, three sessions per day.

■ **Week 2**
PURPOSE: To build strength and endurance

Sitting:

■ Squeeze your pelvic floor muscles for two seconds. Then rest for two seconds. Repeat this ten times, three sessions per day.

■ Squeeze your pelvic floor muscles and hold for ten seconds, then rest for ten seconds. Repeat this ten times, three sessions per day.

■ **Week 3 → Continuing Until Dry**
PURPOSE: To build strength and endurance

Standing:

■ Squeeze your pelvic floor muscles for two seconds. Then rest for two seconds. Repeat this ten times, three sessions per day.

- Squeeze your pelvic floor muscles and hold for ten seconds, then rest for ten seconds. Repeat this ten times, three sessions per day.

- **Week 4 → Continuing Beyond**
  PURPOSE: To coordinate the pelvic floor with other muscles

  Add: Pelvic Floor Plus Accessory Muscle Exercise
  Lying on your back:
  Contract **four** muscles, all at once:

  - Start by contracting your **pelvic floor muscles**.
  - Contract your **transversus abdominus** (deep abdominal core muscle) by bringing your navel to your spine.
  - Squeeze your heels together (to add your **hip adductor muscles**).
  - Squeeze your buttocks together (to add your **gluteal muscles**).
  - Contract each of these muscles, one by one, and then **hold all four** muscles together at the same time for ten seconds. Repeat ten times. Do one set per day.

- **Week 5 → Continuing Beyond**
  PURPOSE: To improve function by adding the pelvic brace to daily activities

  Note: You may read Chapters 4 and 5 if you have urge incontinence and/or urinary urgency, frequency, or nocturia, in addition to stress incontinence.

  Add: Pelvic Brace With Daily Activities
  In various positions throughout the day:

  The pelvic brace combines a pelvic floor contraction with a contraction of the transversus abdominus muscle. Squeeze these **two** muscles together and **hold** them **during** daily life activities such as coughing, sneezing, laughing, standing up from sitting, blowing your nose, lifting, squatting, lunging, climbing/descending stairs, playing sports, or any activity that you do routinely.

- **Week 6 → Continuing Beyond**
  PURPOSE: To improve coordination

<u>Add</u>: Advanced Coordination Exercise for the Pelvic Floor
    Muscles
Sitting on a towel roll:

- Do the *combination exercise*: Squeeze your pelvic floor muscles and hold for five seconds, then quickly squeeze them
  three times with your best effort. The total contraction takes
  ten seconds. Repeat five times, once a day.
- Do the *stair exercise*: Squeeze your pelvic floor muscles for five
  seconds, then relax halfway (not all the way) and hold this
  half-effort contraction for another five seconds. The total contraction takes ten seconds. Repeat five times, once a day.

- **Week 7 → Continuing Beyond**
  PURPOSE: To increase muscle tone
  <u>Add</u>: Advanced Toning Exercises for the Pelvic Floor Muscles
  Standing, and with functional activities:

  Optional: Purchase vaginal weights. Start with the lightest weight
      and progress to the heaviest weight. Strive to hold each
      weight in your vagina for fifteen minutes before pro-
      gressing to the next higher weight, as you improve your
      muscle tone while doing your daily indoor chores.

- **Week 8 → Continuing Beyond**
  PURPOSE: To add resistance

  <u>Add</u>: Advanced Resistance Exercises for the Pelvic Floor
      Muscles
  Lying on your back:

  Optional: Purchase the KegelMaster® device to use at home to
      add resistance to your pelvic floor exercises from Week
      1. Insert vaginally. (Refer to DVD that comes with the
      unit.)

  Super Kegel: Ten 20-second contractions, ten repetitions.
  Glazer's Protocol: 20 minutes of endurance contractions, twice
  a day.

WAY TO GO! You have worked hard and been diligent in your exercise regimen. Are you nearly dry—wearing fewer or no pads? Have you experienced a noticeable difference in your life? We hope so, and we applaud you for taking the necessary steps to make a difference.

Although both of us authors are lovers of fashion, we do not believe diapers are haute couture. What they are, however, is "big business," and their manufacturers are doing whatever it takes to make them more appealing to the ever-growing incontinence market. Don't fall victim to their ploys. Instead, use this program to enjoy your newfound freedom. Keep up with your routine. Use the exercises you learned in your daily life. Continue to work the plan and become a fashion plate all unto yourself.

Do you leak urine on the way to the bathroom? Do you know where every bathroom is in your hometown? Are you losing sleep because of numerous nighttime bathroom visits? These problems are due to an unstable bladder. Now you are ready to put your newfound pelvic floor strength to excellent use, by learning how to retrain your bladder in Chapters 4 and 5.

4 Urge Urinary Incontinence

"POTTY TRAINED": MEET STEPHANIE

Spending her days in and out of the car, dragging her toddler son along from errand to errand, had become routine for Stephanie. What had also become routine was that each time she pulled the car into the garage, the urge to go to the bathroom suddenly hit, and it hit hard. It was like clockwork, but to her surprise the actual time of day was irrelevant: It was the ritual of arriving home that triggered the response: As she made her way into her garage, she just had *to go.*

Stephanie often left three-year-old Tommy strapped in his car seat in the garage while she made a mad dash to the bathroom to relieve herself. This regularly evoked crying and almost always brought on hollers of "Mommmmmmy, let me out!" Her anxiety, escalated by her son's screaming, only made matters worse.

The door that led from the garage into the house was a point of pause, especially if it was locked. Like Pavlov's dog, Stephanie felt the urge to urinate more severely the moment she inserted her key into the lock. Alternating between dancing a jig and keeping her legs crossed in a viselike grip, Stephanie futzed impatiently with the key so she could make it inside.

She didn't always make it. Many days she went from the bathroom to the laundry room, carrying her wet underwear and her shame with her. Even on the best of days she could hear Tommy's trailing voice, "Mommy, where are you?" and "Get me out of here!" Feeling like a fool for wetting her pants, and a bad mother to boot, Stephanie was overwhelmed.

For many mothers, being overwhelmed is part of the job description. What Stephanie didn't know was she shared something besides motherhood with millions of women around the world: urge urinary incontinence. Women who suffer from urge incontinence have bladders that can be provoked by a myriad of cues and circumstances. Any sort of running water usually works. Turning on the washing machine, dishwasher, shower, or sink can be a catalyst for disaster.

The urge to urinate becomes so immediate that some women wet their pants standing right at the toilet. Entering a crowded, public restroom can be a fate worse than death for a woman with urge incontinence, as she groans, "Oh no; there's a line!" Women with urge incontinence cannot wait.

Urge urinary incontinence is defined as an involuntary loss of urine associated with a sudden, strong desire to void (urgency). These are the leaks that happen while en route to the bathroom. Whereas stress incontinence can produce an unwanted dribble of urine caused by a cough or sneeze, urge incontinence is a dam break. Once triggered, the bladder often empties completely.

Urge incontinence is both a physiological and a psychological problem. It is physiological in that the bladder has lost its ability to regulate its urges, and the pelvic floor muscles are not strong enough to keep the urethra closed to prevent leakage. It is also psychological, because the brain sees or hears something that stimulates the need to go to the bathroom and directs the bladder to empty. Soon the woman, like a puppet, has no control over her body, and her bladder is the puppeteer. Her bladder literally starts controlling her life. Fortunately, this dilemma can easily be solved through clinical physical therapy. With this book, you can start the process of healing yourself at home now.

DO I HAVE URINARY URGENCY?

Four common urinary conditions are (a) urinary urgency, (b) urge incontinence, (c) urinary frequency, and (d) nocturia. All of these conditions can make life annoying or downright unbearable, totally affecting the quality of your life, day and night. In all four of these related conditions the bladder gives you uncontrollable urgent signals, often with very little urine in the bladder and no forewarning. These problems are often interrelated and come as a package deal.

As you learned in Chapter 1, there is a natural process to emptying your bladder. The urges you feel are not supposed to be answered with an immediate run to the nearest bathroom; instead, they are just early signals to let your brain know there is urine available to void. You are the owner of your own body and the bladder within it. It is *your* choice to decide when to go to the bathroom. Unfortunately, the order often gets turned around, and hence you can have one or more of the following diagnoses.

With urinary urgency, the bladder becomes overactive and gives sudden, forceful urges that are so strong it is extremely difficult to get to the bathroom in time. Sometimes there are triggers prompting the brain to give the signal to the bladder to contract forcefully, long before you are in the bathroom and ready.

Arriving home is a very common trigger (this is called *key-in-the-door syndrome*). This sudden urge that hits you after arriving home clearly has nothing to do with how much urine is actually in your bladder. Arriving home fifteen minutes earlier or fifteen minutes later would have triggered the same violent need to use the bathroom. If you make it to the bathroom in time after a sudden, uncontrollable urge to urinate, then you have urinary urgency. In severe cases, urinating doesn't even help, and the feeling of urgency remains strong all day long.

Other urge triggers include cold weather and nervousness. Unfortunately, many women with this condition live their lives in a constant state of anxiety.

DO I HAVE URGE URINARY INCONTINENCE?

If, after feeling strong urinary urgency, you *do not* make it to the bathroom in time, then you have urge urinary incontinence, which stems from the same underlying problem as urinary urgency: The overactive bladder doesn't wait for any signal from you, such as the "letting go" of the pelvic floor muscles, to relay that you are ready. The bladder seems to have a mind of its own and empties fully, defying the owner of this bladder—*you*—as you are trying to, for example, grocery shop, or watch a movie. These accidents of urge incontinence are often huge in volume, because the entire bladder empties, and they are devastatingly hard to cover up.

DO I HAVE URINARY FREQUENCY?

Urinary frequency is when you urinate an excessive number of times during the day, driven to the bathroom by your bladder. If your frequency is severe, you may feel the need to urinate all day long, and you may use the bathroom as often as every thirty to sixty minutes. Do you feel as though you live with one toe in the bathroom?

What is normal? What is excessive urination? It is considered normal to empty the bladder every three to four hours. This translates to a total of five to seven times within a twenty-four hour period. This becomes the goal of physical therapy.

The bladder's job is to store urine. Ideally, it empties only on the request of the person. However, because it is susceptible to other triggers, your bladder can fall into the bad habit of needing to be relieved an inordinately high number of times. A frequency problem, which develops as a common side effect of having a urinary tract infection (UTI), can linger long after the infection is resolved. A pregnant woman's bladder needs to be emptied more frequently, because of the pressure from the fetus, and sometimes this sensation hasn't yet ended even when the child is old enough to vote!

Many women go so often—up to every half-hour—that they complain they are living their lives in the bathroom, and they are. Don't let your frequency get this bad. If it already is, this book will fix it. How can you shop, get errands done, see a movie, take a car trip, play bridge, or visit a museum if you need to visit the bathroom this often? You can't.

Have you ever *intentionally* gone too often (termed *just-in-case voiding*) as a way to ward off your leakage by trying to keep the bladder empty? This strategy rarely works. The bladder is never empty. Shortly after post-void hand washing is complete, the kidneys have probably made another two ounces of urine, so your ability to leak is always there. By voiding too often on purpose, you inadvertently create a constant need to go to the bathroom. Your bladder gets used to being emptied every hour, so it forgets how to stretch and hold more. Pretty soon your bladder starts giving you the urge-to-go signal earlier and earlier, and before long you will develop a genuine frequency problem.

Don't take vital social activities out of your life, giving half-truths as excuses about why you can't attend them. Instead, work with us and this book to reduce your frequency so you can live your life to the fullest.

DO I HAVE NOCTURIA?

Nocturia is urinary frequency that happens during the sleeping hours. Even though you are not drinking, and your metabolism is slower while you are resting overnight, an overactive bladder gives you no rest, literally. Getting up once to use the bathroom is considered normal for a senior adult. It is not considered normal for a young to middle-aged woman, who shouldn't need to get up at all. In severe cases of nocturia, women rise four to six times per night to go to the bathroom, night after night, year after year. They are living their lives in a sleep-deprived state, which unnecessarily robs them of energy, memory, and mental alertness.

A study conducted by researchers at the National Association for Continence on 1,111 middle-aged American women demonstrated that not getting enough sleep (due to nocturia) disrupted women's sense of normalcy and negatively affected their quality of life (Levkowicz, Whitmore, & Muller, 2011). We look into the value of sleep for our overall health in the next chapter. Furthermore, women with nocturia were more likely to report being depressed than those without nocturia. (We explore the double syndrome of depression and incontinence in more detail in Chapter 9.) On the basis of these findings, the authors of this study strongly urged primary care and specialty physicians to address nocturia during regular office visits and present all treatment options to their patients (Levkowicz et al., 2011). The real shame about nocturia is that too many women suffer needlessly, because it is totally correctable.

WHAT CAUSES URGE URINARY INCONTINENCE AND FREQUENCY?

There is no exact cause of urge urinary incontinence, frequency, urgency, and nocturia. The medical diagnostic name for these conditions—*detrusor instability*—describes them well. This means that the detrusor muscle (i.e., your bladder) is unstable or overactive. Your bladder is a very receptive organ, and it doesn't take much for it to develop bad habits. Although there is no definite cause for frequency and urge incontinence, there are known contributing factors, and they are primarily *behavioral* in nature; for example, perhaps when you had a baby you got out of bed twice every night to breastfeed. Despite the fact that your son is now a high school quarterback, you are still arising from bed twice nightly to empty your bladder, perpetuating your nocturia. Or perhaps you developed a UTI a year ago, and although the pain and burning are gone, your too-frequent bathrooms trips still plague you. You will learn all about UTIs in the next section.

In addition to the physical discomfort, there is a definite mental stress component to urgency and urge incontinence as well. Knowing you have arrived home will invariably trigger a mad dash to the bathroom, as it did with Stephanie. Worrying about the possibility of needing to find a bathroom while running errands will certainly cause you to map out all the available clean restrooms in your hometown. This much attention paid to your bladder will definitely get it talking to you! All you probably need to do is *think* about going, and the urge comes on. This is because the brain is part of the reflex that causes you to urinate.

Diet also can provoke urgency and incontinence. Dietary bladder irritants, such as the caffeine in coffee, tea, and many cola drinks; acidic fruit juices, such as orange juice; and alcohol all provoke urgency, leading to incontinence. When you say, "Iced tea goes right through me," what you are really saying is that the caffeine in tea acts as a bladder irritant, provoking an urgency to urinate. (A more comprehensive listing of other dietary irritants, and their substitutes, is provided in the next chapter, on page 115.)

Despite how easily the bladder adopts bad habits, it also is a very *re*trainable organ! In the next chapter you will learn to make behavioral changes that will enable *you* to choose when to empty your bladder. Imagine how nice it will feel not to think about your bladder issues 24/7, as you overcome your urge incontinence.

Unfortunately, just when Stephanie thought the embarrassment and aggravation of wetting her own pants couldn't get any worse, it did. Stephanie went through three to four pairs of underwear a day. Sadly, she often had to deal with the wetness for awhile, if her urge incontinence hit while she was out of the house or if she had to tend to Tommy's needs first. She did wear pads, but with the amount of urine she would release, the pad was often saturated.

As a result, she found herself with one UTI after another. She was so ashamed to admit to her doctor the real reason she needed yet another prescription for antibiotics that she lied to him when he asked her about it, claiming she had no idea why the UTIs kept occurring. The higher need to use the bathroom more often, during the burning sensation of the UTI, made her frequency and urge urinary incontinence worse to boot.

UTIs commonly occur in association with urinary incontinence and can actually be the underlying cause of urgency, frequency, and urge urinary incontinence. UTIs are a less-than-pleasant condition, to say the least. Most women will experience one at some point in their lives. As a topic most of us will gloss over in the doctor's office, many of us might not be aware of how some of our everyday habits are the origins of this uncomfortable problem. We apologize in advance for any uneasiness the information presented in the next section might create: Get ready for an eye-opening education.

UNDERSTANDING URINARY TRACT INFECTIONS

As the name implies, UTIs are infections of the urinary tract, and most occur in the lower urinary tract, which comprises the bladder and urethra (the tube through which urine leaves the body). About ninety percent of UTIs are caused by *Escherichia coli* (*E. coli*) bacteria. *E. coli* lives abundantly in the rectum (where bowel movements leave the body), but when these bacteria migrate into the urethra, a UTI can develop. The female anatomy makes all women susceptible to UTIs because of the short distance between the urethra and the rectum. Half of all women will develop a UTI at some time in their lives. Add a urine-saturated pad to the equation and you now have the warm, dark, moist environment in which bacteria thrive. Thus, incontinent women are inherently at a higher risk of developing UTIs.

How do you know you have a UTI? Symptoms include a burning sensation when urinating; cloudy or odorous urine; and a strong urge to urinate that causes you to pass frequent, small amounts of urine. In fact, having a UTI can be the root cause of urinary frequency, which can last for years after the infection has resolved. Your doctor diagnoses a UTI through a urinalysis of your urine sample. Normally, urine is sterile, so having bacteria in your urine is abnormal and thus helps diagnose a UTI.

In most UTIs, *E. coli* bacteria have somehow, someway, made their way from the rectal area to the urethral area. How does this happen? By far, the most common time when bacteria are spread from the anal region to the urethral region is after a bowel movement. Fecal matter is loaded with *E. coli*. Just wiping from the front to the back, like our mothers told us is, frankly, not good enough. You also should clean the entire rectal area with soap and water after every bowel movement and continue wiping front to back with soft toilet tissue until the tissue is clean and odorless or, better yet, shower to get fully clean after your bowel movements—without a washcloth, which spreads germs. It is too bad the European bidet never became a mainstream bathroom fixture in America. One easy way to manage the wiping issue is to use personal cleansing wipes at home or on the go.

Improper underwear selection and laundry methods also can be contributing factors to developing a UTI. Thong underwear creates a "clothesline" effect, allowing rectal bacteria to "crawl" to the urethra. Fuller coverage, cotton underpants that you change once or even twice a day are preferable. Do not wash your outer clothes, towels, or rags with your underpants. Wash your underpants separately. Laundry soap is not a perfect germ killer, especially in cold water. Use hot water and bleach, if possible, for a better disinfectant effect.

Women who are sexually active tend to get more UTIs, because germs can travel more easily between the rectum and the urethra during physical contact. Be extra cautious with the vaginal-entry-from-behind position during sexual intercourse ("doggie" style). It is advisable to drink a full glass of water and urinate soon after intercourse to help flush out bacteria that may have attached themselves to the lining of the urethra before an infection can develop.

Cranberry juice has been found to help treat and prevent UTIs. The sugars found in cranberry juice coat the lining of the urethra, making it harder for *E. coli* to stick and cause an infection. CranActin is a brand of cranberry juice in pill form.

Even better is a simple sugar called D-Mannose that, some people claim, works fifty times better than cranberry juice while being essentially the same method of prevention. If you are prone to chronic UTIs, take a low dose of D-Mannose (e.g., 1,000 mg once a day), because long-term use is perfectly safe (Wright and Lenard, 2001). (We provide dose recommendations in the next section.) Take a larger dose of D-Mannose (e.g., 1,000 mg six times a day) at the first sign of infection. Please discuss this with your physician first before replacing your antibiotic regimen with D-Mannose. It is not uncommon for antibiotics to stop working in some women after repeated, long-term use, so your doctor may welcome your suggestion of a more natural approach. You will also avoid one of the most common side effects of antibiotics: a reactive yeast infection, which occurs as the bacterial balance in the vagina is altered and the yeast multiplies unchecked. Because neither cranberry juice nor D-Mannose actually kills bacteria, a yeast infection does not take place.

The good news is that some common-sense changes can make a big difference in preventing future UTIs. In this final section, we provide a list of thirty practical behavioral tips to help you prevent your next UTI.

YOUR HOME PROGRAM:

30 WAYS TO PREVENT URINARY TRACT INFECTIONS

1. Wash your rectal area with soap and water and soft toilet paper after every bowel movement. Keep cleaning and drying until the toilet paper is clean and odor-free, or shower after your bowel movements.
2. Use natural, nonperfumed soap.
3. Wash your hands often.
4. Wash towels after every use—a hand towel for your private area saves laundry.
5. Drink cranberry juice or take CranActin.
6. Take D-Mannose. At the first sign of a UTI, take 1,000 mg, six times a day, with six ounces of water. On Day 2, take 1,000 mg, four times a day, with six ounces of water. On Day 3, take 1,000 mg, three times a day, with six ounces of water. For preventative maintenance, take 1,000 mg, once a day, with 6 ounces of water. D-Mannose is available in either pill or powder form. (See Appendix IV, page 251, for discount ordering information.)
7. Clean your rectal and genital areas with soap and water before sexual intercourse.
8. Drink a full glass of water and urinate directly after sexual intercourse.
9. Be extra cautious with the vaginal-entry-from-behind position during sexual intercourse ("doggie" style).
10. Change menstrual pads and incontinence pads often, to minimize creating the ideal environment for germs (i.e., warm, dark, moist).
11. Change your underwear every day, or even twice a day, if you are moist from vaginal discharge or urinary leakage.
12. Wash your underwear separately from outer clothes, towels, and rags. Wash your underwear separately in hot water, with bleach if possible.

13. Step into your underwear without touching the crotch area with the bottom of your feet. Always put your shoes on after your underwear, even at the gym.

14. Never put underwear back on once it has been on the floor, or on your pet's favorite couch or spot on your bed.

15. Hand-wash your bathing suit with soap after every use, especially the crotch area (even if you didn't swim).

16. Wear only cotton underpants—no nylon or rayon—for better breathability.

17. Don't wear thongs. They create a direct line from rectum to urethra, potentially transmitting *E. coli.*

18. Make sure underwear is the proper size, big enough to allow air circulation.

19. At night, wear cotton pajamas or nightgowns without underwear to improve airflow.

20. Take a shower every day. The ideal time to take your shower is after a bowel movement.

21. Do not take baths; water-borne germs can float from the rectum to the urethra. If you want to take a soaking, relaxation bath, you could shower or do a sponge bath before, in order to pre-clean your rectal area.

22. Do not use washcloths; they spread germs between body parts. If you must, use a separate, freshly laundered washcloth on your urethral, vaginal, and rectal areas—in that order!

23. Avoid douches, deodorant sprays, or other feminine products that can irritate the urethra.

24. Never wear pantyhose and long pants together, because this limits air flow to your genital area.

25. Don't wear jeans or other pants that are too tight and rub in the crotch area.

26. Eat a well-balanced diet rich in antioxidants to reduce inflammation.

27. Eat yogurt, especially brands with probiotics, such as Activia.

28. Minimize acidic juices, such as orange juice and grapefruit juice. Grape and apple juice are less irritating to the urethra.

29. Try drinking low-acid coffee. Trader Joe's (http://www.trader joes.com) carries low-acid coffee beans.

30. Minimize your alcohol intake. Alcohol is very irritating to the bladder and urethra.

How many of these behavioral changes should you make in order to better prevent UTIs? This is up to you. Photocopy this list and use a highlighter on the changes you want to make. Many of these suggestions are simple, but powerful, and they make so much sense. UTIs are preventable!

You now have learned about urge urinary incontinence and its variations. Were you able to identify your own type? Sadly, urge urinary incontinence is hard to cover up because it can mean emptying your entire bladder, creating a much larger leak than a pad can handle, causing your outer clothes to become wet. Unlike stress urinary incontinence, which can often involve just a few drops, urge urinary incontinence leaks can be huge. Obviously, urge incontinence can leave you wet and uncomfortable and possibly lead to a UTI, a miserable accompaniment to your incontinence.

In this chapter we have given you some simple yet powerful tools to help modify your behaviors and habits in an effort to prevent future UTIs. Making some or all of these changes in your normal routine will dramatically reduce your susceptibility to UTIs.

Let's say your UTI is now gone. Your frequency, nocturia, urgency, and urge urinary incontinence remain. Now what? In the next chapter, we give you the answers. You will meet a woman who suffers not only from urge urinary incontinence but also from the demoralizing side effects associated with it. You will see how she takes charge of her life and her bladder, and very soon you will be making these changes too.

"If nothing ever changed, there'd be no butterflies."
—Author unknown

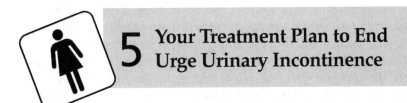

5 Your Treatment Plan to End Urge Urinary Incontinence

"THE HOMEBODY": MEET EMILY

I rarely leave my house. The good news is, for my age—seventy-three—I am quite a "techie!" I can find my way around the Internet better than most college students can. I even text my grandkids! I used to be very active and have always been interested in the latest trends or next big thing. That is probably why I got interested in computers in the first place. Now, staying at home, social networks like Facebook have become my lifeline to the outside world.

I do everything online. I buy my groceries and pet supplies that way, and I have my prescriptions mailed to me. I visit a few chat rooms and play bridge on the computer. The bad news, of course, is that I am a virtual prisoner in my own home. I am certainly of sound mind; it's the body part that has been letting me down.

It wasn't always like this. I used to be busy and involved in the community. I was a member of the city garden club, played cards with friends in a bridge club, and loved to try different restaurants and see movies with my husband. Unfortunately, one day at the garden club my private problem became a very public one.

I was working at my plot alongside many other friends who maintained spaces in the city's community garden. I was filling my watering can when a sudden strong urge came on, and I started wetting my pants. I couldn't stop going, so I quickly spilled some of the water out of my can onto myself to mask my accident. My friends teased me for being such a klutz, but luckily they didn't guess the true reason for the wet spot. I had had problems like this before, when I didn't make it to the bathroom in time, but they were much milder and usually happened at night. Leakages started happening more and more during the day and, unfortunately, I didn't always have a watering can handy. I usually had a clever excuse, but it was getting increasingly harder to cover up.

I had to figure out a way to deal with the problem. I had worn sanitary pads for years, but more recently I had resorted to diapers. Although they were expensive, they seemed to work pretty well, and I was determined not to give up my outings. But then everything changed for the worse.

Between hands at one of my bridge club games, I stood up to use the bathroom. The movement caused a little trickle to begin leaking into my pad. That was normal and OK because I also had on my hot but trustworthy diaper. You see, I wear a pad on top of the diaper in order to get more use out of the diaper. But I also had a much bigger problem.

Embarrassingly, urine was not the only thing that leaked out that time: Along with my urine dribble, I felt the pressure of a gas bubble in my rectal area. I tried to hold it back, but couldn't, and as I stood up the gas emerged as well. Suddenly the room was potent with an awful smell, and a very uncomfortable silence flooded the room. I walked, red faced, to the guest bathroom.

As the odor evaporated, so did my spirit. I finished the game that day, but I never went back. I gave different feeble excuses each week. One week, it was a "doctor's appointment." Another week, it was "a repairman I had to meet at the house." It went on like that for about a month, and then I gave up the bridge club altogether, and the garden club, too.

Soon I started having my groceries delivered, and I even gave up dining out with my husband. The urinating problem was one thing, but the gas was beyond resolve. Almost every time I had a urine leak, gas would release as well. One by one, I slowly began taking social activities out of my life.

That sadly brings me to where I am today: depressed and living a pretty pathetic existence. As long as I don't venture too far from my bathroom, I am OK. My husband is aware of my incontinence issue and tries to be empathic. We have never openly discussed my gas problem, but I am sure he knows—he would have to. It is one subject that I am too ashamed to discuss with anyone, even him. The only complaint he does have is that his sleep is constantly interrupted by my three bathroom visits every night. He has suggested separate bedrooms, and unfortunately, that may be inevitable. Then I will feel even more isolated.

If Chapter 3 is the "heart" of this book for stress incontinence, this chapter is the "soul" for urge incontinence. The solutions we present in this chapter will capitalize on your newfound pelvic floor strength and change your life in ways you never thought possible, day and night. You will enjoy more freedom to lead the active, worry-free life you desire and deserve. This knowledge will enable you to kick your bladder into the back seat where it belongs, putting *you* back in the driver's seat, exercising full control over your bladder.

As with Stephanie from Chapter 4, Emily suffers from urge urinary incontinence, the second most common form of incontinence. Furthermore, Emily suffers from a combination of three types of incontinence. She has both urge and stress incontinence (also referred to as *mixed incontinence*), plus gas incontinence. Poor Emily feels disheartened and ashamed.

Emily's sleep deprivation, which is due to multiple nighttime bathroom trips, recently caused her daughter to question her sanity. Emily couldn't remember her own birth date when she was filling out a form. Her daughter forced her to schedule a checkup with her general practitioner. That visit changed everything.

Although Emily was there to discuss memory loss and constant fatigue, the doctor asked her about her sleep patterns. She reluctantly admitted to her nightly bathroom visits and went on to confess her incontinence problem. She expressed her overwhelming sadness and her dreaded fear of another accident in public. In response, the doctor recommended bladder retraining through physical therapy.

BLADDER RETRAINING

Luckily, the bladder is a very trainable organ. In this chapter you will learn physical therapy behavioral modification techniques and exercises to retrain your bladder back to normalcy; however, before your bladder retraining can begin, you will need much information, because the process is highly individualized. The types of information you will need include the following:

- The quantities and types of food and drink you consume (to analyze hydration and spot bladder irritants in your diet)
- How often and how much you urinate (to analyze your frequency)
- How much you leak and how often you have leakage (to assess the severity of your urinary incontinence)
- Which physical activities provoke your leakage (to determine whether you have stress, urge, or mixed urinary incontinence)

- Whether you have an urge with either the voids or the leakage (to distinguish urgency versus urge incontinence versus just-in-case voiding)
- The number of pads or diapers you use per day (to quantify your problem)

This is a lot of necessary information! You will need to fill out a Daily Voiding Diary (also called a *Bladder Diary* or *Bladder Log*; see Appendix II, page 245). Without such a diary, you probably have no idea how many trips to the bathroom you actually take, how much you drink, or how many times you have leakage per day.

This first step in the bladder retraining process gives you a snapshot of your eating, drinking, leakage, and voiding habits. With your diary of data, you can begin to analyze the severity of your problem and use the tools provided in this home program to create a bladder retraining plan that is right for you.

If you are already working with a physical therapist, you may have a voiding diary. If you are not yet working with a physical therapist, you should complete a voiding diary, because it will provide valuable information to share with the physical therapist as she assists in your treatment. Ideally, this voiding diary is filled out before your first visit to the physical therapist, or it is given as homework at the first visit.

Turn to the Daily Voiding Diary on page 245 in the back of this book and make an *enlarged* copy of the Daily Voiding Diary provided therein. The copy should be full-page size, to make it easy to record your data. We understand that filling out a voiding diary is a bit of a hassle. This is not an exercise done in vain, though, because you will learn a lot about your own bladder habits. Some of the details may surprise you!

This mandatory first step will launch the process of owning a bladder that no longer holds you captive. The sooner you complete your diary, the easier it will be for your physical therapist to help you, and for you to help yourself.

FILL OUT A VOIDING DIARY TODAY!

Turn to the Daily Voiding Diary (page 245 in the back of the book) and make several *enlarged* copies of it. Fill out your data for a twenty-four-hour period. Take this first step in identifying your personal bladder issues.

We provide full instructions on how to fill out a voiding diary in the next section. You will also see an example of one already completed, by Emily.

YOUR HOME PROGRAM: HOW TO COMPLETE A VOIDING DIARY

You Will Need

Daily Voiding Diary (page 245, copied and enlarged)
A sixteen-ounce measuring cup, a watch, and a pen

Column 1: The rows in this column comprise one day, a twenty-four-hour period, starting with 12:00 midnight. Use the nearest hour or the half-hour (use the line between the hours to indicate when something took place as it pertains to Columns 2 through 6).

Column 2: List all the different foods you eat this day. Write down the types and amounts (in ounces) of all beverages you drink. Record each menu item across from the time of day that you consumed it.

Column 3: When you go to the bathroom, you will need to urinate into a 16-ounce measuring cup. You do not have to throw the measuring cup away afterward; just clean it thoroughly. Remember, urine is sterile! Measure each amount voided in ounces, dump the urine into the toilet, and flush. Record this amount by writing the number of ounces that you urinated across from the appropriate time on the form. (Include the bathroom trips for bowel movements; estimating the ounces of these voids is OK.) Later you can count out your voids in seconds, instead of measuring in ounces. Most women urinate about an ounce per second, and it is much more convenient to measure in seconds.

Column 4: When you have a leakage of urine, rate it as S (small: just a drop or two), M (medium: the amount wets your underwear), or L (large: the amount wets your outerwear or the floor). Enter S/M/L across from the time that the leakage took place. If you wear pads, estimate accordingly.

Column 5: This column relates to Columns 3 and 4. Was there an urge sensation when you used the bathroom or had some leakage? In Column 3 or 4, write "Yes" or "No" at the time of day that corresponds to your entry.

Column 6: Across from the leak you listed in Column 4, state the activity that caused the leak. Was it coughing, sneezing, lifting, standing up, washing dishes, or urgency on arriving home? If you don't know what caused the leakage, leave it blank.

Bottom: Here you record your name, date, bodyweight, and number (and types) of pads used.

Learning how to use a form is always easier after you see one that has been filled out correctly. Take a look at the next page, which shows a completed voiding diary that Emily filled out.

As we know, Emily is a seventy-three-year-old woman who suffers with mixed urinary incontinence. She also has urinary urgency, urinary frequency, nocturia, and gas incontinence. She has had these problems for more than thirty years. She was suffering in silence until she finally spoke up to her family practice physician, who promptly referred her for physical therapy.

After we analyze Emily's problems by going over her voiding diary, we will explain how she should retrain her bladder, make dietary changes, and rehabilitate her pelvic floor muscles in order to get rid of her incontinence. Let's learn from her poor bladder habits as she gives us concrete examples of the conditions described in Chapter 4.

ANALYZING A VOIDING DIARY

Did you complete your one-day voiding diary yet? If you have not done so, it is imperative that you do it soon. The information in his chapter will make much more sense if you can *apply* it directly to *yourself*.

In the meantime, you can tell a lot just by looking at Emily's one-day voiding diary on the next page. In the sections that follow, we identify and discuss all of Emily's problems, one by one. As we do this, consider which symptoms *you* may have. No two diaries are alike, and in this chapter we provide the general advice you will need to apply to your own situation.

DAILY VOIDING DIARY

Column 1	Column 2	Column 3	Column 4	Column 5	Column 6
Time of Day	INTAKE: TYPE of Food TYPE and AMOUNT of Beverages in Ounces	Amount Voided in Toilet: • In Ounces OR • In Seconds	Amount of Leakage: S / M / L	Was an Urge Present? Yes / No	Which Activities Caused Leakage?
MIDNIGHT					
1:00 AM		2 oz		yes	
2:00 AM					
3:00 AM		1 oz	L	yes – @ toilet	
4:00 AM					
5:00 AM		2 oz		yes	
6:00 AM	8 oz Caffeinated				
7:00 AM	Coffee, 8 oz O.J.	2 oz		yes	
8:00 AM	Oatmeal	1 oz	M	yes – on way	
9:00 AM		2 oz		yes	to toilet
10:00 AM		~2 oz (w BM)		no	
11:00 AM		1 oz		yes	
NOON	8 oz Water, Sandwich	1 oz		yes	
1:00 PM	Baked Beans		L		arriving
2:00 PM		4 oz		yes	home
3:00 PM	8 oz Water, apple, cheese	2 oz		no	
4:00 PM		1 oz	S (Gas too)	no – Lifting	groceries
5:00 PM	8 oz Wine, Lasagna				
6:00 PM	Broccoli, Salad	3 oz		yes	
7:00 PM		1 oz		yes	
8:00 PM	8 oz Water, sugar-free	1 oz		yes	
9:00 PM	Candy	1 oz	L	yes – Doing	
10:00 PM		1 oz		no	Dishes
11:00 PM	TO BED →	2 oz		yes	

Body weight: __160__ lbs.   TYPE & NUMBER of pads used today: _5 medium pads + 2 Diapers_

NAME: ___Emily___   DATE:_____

Emily's daily voiding diary.

Pad Usage

Emily's mixed incontinence is moderate to severe. She is using an average of two diapers per day, one for daytime and one for sleeping. They are expensive, so she also places a pad on top of the diaper so she can change just the pad throughout the day, saving the diaper if she can. She used five medium, stick-on incontinence pads this particular day in addition to the two diapers, totaling seven products per day. Changing her pad often helps prevent the urine odor and keeps the diaper rash at a minimum, so she tries to change the pad every time she wets it. She has found what she refers to as a "lifesaver" in multi-use Desitin® for her diaper rash. It is a clear formula that coats and protects her, without leaving her smelling like a baby. She hates to admit her incontinence is worsening, but her escalating pad usage is the proof.

Poor Hydration

Emily weighs 160 lbs but only drinks a total of 48 ounces of fluids in a day. She should be drinking about 80 ounces of fluid for her size. She (erroneously) thinks that if she drinks less, she will leak less. This is a misconception; usually just the opposite is true. Poor hydration results in dark, concentrated, smelly urine that is more acidic and irritating to the bladder than clearer urine. An irritated bladder gives stronger and more frequent urges than it otherwise would. Urine should be just slightly yellow in color. Thus, Emily's poor hydration and dark urine have actually caused *more* urgency, frequency, and leakage—just the opposite of what she was trying to achieve. (We discuss proper hydration and diet later in this chapter.)

Bladder Irritants

Emily drinks caffeinated coffee as well as orange juice and alcohol, which are the three biggest bladder irritants, and indeed, they have caused increased bladder urgency and frequency in Emily.

Bowel Irritants

Emily likes chocolate, but she eats a sugar-free type to save calories. Unfortunately, the ingredients used in sugar-free candies and baked goods can cause severe intestinal cramping and significant amounts of gas. She also eats a lot of broccoli and beans, other notorious producers of gas.

Urinary Frequency

Emily urinated eighteen times in the twenty-four-hour period depicted in previous page, instead of the normal five to seven times.

She has a severe frequency problem. Understandably, all of her voids are small in volume (one to four ounces each). She uses the bathroom approximately every hour instead of holding her urine for three to four hours. Her bladder is not storing urine well at all. Emily worries incessantly about where the closest bathroom is. In her hometown, she knows the location of every public restroom. This is called *bathroom mapping*. The problem is compounded when Emily travels out of town to an unfamiliar place. The anxiety of not knowing where the bathrooms are in unfamiliar locales makes her urgency and frequency worse. Sometimes she rationalizes that it's easier to just stay home.

Nocturia

Every night, like clockwork, Emily gets out of bed three times to use the bathroom; in other words, her bladder wakes her up every two hours. Because she never sleeps more than two hours at a time, she rarely enters the deep rapid eye movement (REM) sleep stage, which is one of the most beneficial stages of sleep. This bladder-induced sleep deprivation causes her to have a poor memory and sluggish word recall, and it requires her to take a midday nap to prevent irritability. Some days she admits to being unable to focus, and she turns down social events because of ongoing fatigue. Emily would love to exercise but lacks the energy for it. She feels trapped by her bladder and depressed over the poor quality of her life.

Emily is on an antidepressant, a category of medication that is known to selectively prevent REM sleep, further compounding her sleep deprivation status. Emily is just a shadow of the vibrant woman she once was. Her family gives her behavior another name: *dementia*. They worry she may be showing early signs of Alzheimer's disease. (We explain the negative effects of sleep deprivation later in this chapter.)

Urinary Urgency

Emily states that, out of her eighteen total voids, fourteen of them were accompanied by strong urgency, way out of proportion to the small amount of urine in her bladder (one to four ounces). She made it to the bathroom most of the time. Four times she did not. The bladder holds 16 ounces, but Emily's bladder never gets close to being full.

Stress Urinary Incontinence

Emily had one small leak that was associated with the physical stress of lifting groceries at 4:00 p.m. She noted on her Daily Voiding Diary that some gas escaped with this activity as well.

Urge Urinary Incontinence

Emily had four accidental leaks when she did not make it to the bathroom in time. She had three large leakage episodes when her whole bladder contracted and fully emptied while she was racing to the bathroom, totally out of control. This occurred in the middle of the night, at 3:00 a.m., when she was arriving home from shopping at 1:00 p.m., and while she was washing the dinner dishes at 9:00 p.m. She had one other medium leak at 8:00 a.m., while on the way to the bathroom in the morning.

Gas Incontinence

Emily could not counteract the gaseous pressure she felt when she was lifting her groceries, and gas incontinence was the result, accompanied by stress incontinence.

Just-in-Case Voiding

According to her diary, Emily used the bathroom three times without a need to urinate, going "just in case." She emptied her bladder before leaving the house and again when arriving at her destinations. She admitted that she often tries to keep her bladder empty so she will leak less, although this technique does not seem to be working at all. Instead, it has only been making her frequency problem worse.

The following is a concise list of all of Emily's many diagnoses, as evidenced by her voiding diary:

- **Mixed urinary incontinence:** One episode of stress incontinence plus four episodes of urge incontinence. Urge incontinence is the primary problem in Emily's case.
- **Gas incontinence:** Once per day
- **Severe frequency problem:** Eighteen trips to the bathroom per day
- **Severe urgency problem:** Fourteen times throughout the day
- **Moderate nocturia:** Three trips to the bathroom during the night
- **Sleep deprivation:** Caused by the nocturia

- **Pad dependency:** Two diapers and five medium pads, promoting diaper rash
- **Just-in-case voiding:** Three times per day
- **Poor hydration:** 48 ounces of daily fluid intake; this should be 80 ounces of fluid per day. (See the "DIET AND HYDRATION PLAN" section on page 112 for the ideal fluid-intake formula.)
- **Bladder irritants in diet:** Caffeinated coffee, orange juice, and alcohol
- **Bowel irritants in diet:** Beans, broccoli, and sugar-free candy

Now take out *your* filled-out Daily Voiding Diary (from Appendix II, page 245). Is it a good representation of a normal day? If not, you can certainly fill out a second one on another day. Go through all of the preceding categories and analyze your own diary. Which of the issues just listed do *you* have? Stress incontinence? Urge incontinence? Mixed incontinence? Frequency and nocturia? Are you going "just in case"? How heavy is your pad usage?

ANALYZE YOUR VOIDING DIARY

How much time passes between each trip to the bathroom? Exactly what triggers your leakage: physical activity, beverages, running water, arriving home? Do you have nocturia? Decide whether you have stress, urge, or mixed urinary incontinence. How many leaks are you having per day? How many pads are you using? Make a list of *your* bladder issues that need fixing!

Once you have made your list of urinary problems, you can proceed to the next section and learn how to get rid of them and *retrain* your bladder back to normalcy. Don't throw your first voiding diary away, because you will want to keep it as a memento of the "old" you! Let's create the "new" you and get your life back!

YOUR HOME PROGRAM: HOW TO RETRAIN YOUR BLADDER

Let's continue with Emily's treatment as our example. We chose to highlight Emily's case because she has *every* bladder control issue readers will face. Naturally, not everyone has every problem, as

Emily does; however, pay special attention to the advice given to Emily if you are experiencing the same type of problem. By applying the bladder retraining techniques you will learn in this chapter, you will rid yourself of urge incontinence, urgency, frequency, nocturia, and/or sleep deprivation.

The first phase of Emily's recovery was to learn how to find, isolate, strengthen, condition, and coordinate her pelvic floor muscles with the aid of SEMG or another form of biofeedback, which we discussed at length in Chapter 2.

In accordance with Chapter 3, Emily followed her at-home regimen to strengthen her pelvic floor muscles, and in about five weeks she felt ready for bladder retraining. Most women follow a similar pattern, especially if their abnormal bladder function has been going on for years.

WHEN TO START RETRAINING YOUR BLADDER

You may begin retraining your bladder as soon as your pelvic floor muscles are strong enough to counteract your Herculean bladder muscle. For most women, this is about four weeks into the plan as prescribed in Chapter 3. Please be advised that starting earlier than three to four weeks can be a recipe for failure. By waiting four weeks, you can begin treating your urge incontinence while you continue treating your stress incontinence, building more pelvic floor strength; thus, you will be following along with Chapter 3 and Chapter 5 simultaneously.

After rehabilitating her pelvic floor, Emily can use this new-found strength to begin treating her urge urinary incontinence. She is in dire need of bladder retraining through behavioral modification.

Emily's physical therapist begins this training process by asking Emily to use the bathroom *every hour*. This should be easy for Emily, because she is going that often already. Emily empties her bladder at hourly intervals, even if she does not feel the need to do so. This teaches Emily's bladder how to empty normally, as we described in Chapter 1, initiated not by her bladder but by her "letting go." It also teaches her overactive bladder to relax and depend on her to empty it routinely.

HOW TO START YOUR BLADDER RETRAINING

The process of bladder retraining will vary from woman to woman. If you are currently using the bathroom, let's say, every two hours, then this is where you will start. Use daily diaries to empty your bladder every two hours, even if you *do not feel the need* to go. Your bladder must learn some structure and to rely on your consistency.

On her next visit, one week later, Emily's physical therapist looks at her new Daily Voiding Diary sheets and requests that Emily increase the interval between voids to one and a half hours, because it is getting easier to delay her urinations.

Emily's bladder responds well to this increase, and has even less leakage, so she is progressed to voiding every two hours in her third week. This bladder retraining continues, week by week, until Emily reaches a normal spacing of three to four hours between trips to the bathroom. Usually thirty minutes is added to the interval every week, but if some weeks seem too difficult, two weeks can elapse before widening the interval. Emily's bladder needs some time to perform its intended role in life: storing urine.

HOW TO PROGRESS DURING RETRAINING

Every week you will *add thirty minutes* to your interval, so, if you started with two hours between trips to the bathroom, you will progress to two and a half hours in your second week and then to three hours in your third week. Then you will maintain the interval at between three and four hours, because now you have achieved *normal* bladder function!

What happens, however, if one of those devastatingly strong urges hits before it is time to go, according to your schedule? Thankfully, the physical therapist teaches Emily some very successful techniques from which everyone can benefit.

Urge suppression techniques actually stop the urgency feeling, without using the bathroom. Emily finds this hard to believe. She is very skeptical that these techniques will work on her strong urges and overactive bladder. She is amazed when they do work to actually *turn off* her bladder *without* emptying it!

Whereas relaxing (letting go of) the pelvic floor muscles makes urination start, the reverse is also true. Strong pelvic floor muscle contractions (squeezing) stop the bladder from contracting, making the urge and leakage threats disappear. This is because of a reciprocal reflex in our bodies, called *Bradley's Loop III*. Many of our muscles work in tandem this way, allowing one muscle to contract while the other one relaxes, in an either–or relationship.

For example, if you straighten your knee, your quadricep muscles will contract and shorten, while your hamstring muscles stretch and elongate. When you bend your knee, your hamstring muscles will contract and shorten while your quadricep muscles stretch and elongate. This vice versa effect allows paired muscles to contract reciprocally. Similarly, either the bladder muscle *or* the pelvic floor muscles contract, but not both at the same time. This gives us the control we need.

Because the brain is part of the problem (e.g., when it "knows" it has arrived at home), it also needs to be part of the solution. Mind distraction techniques can allow you to stop thinking of going to the bathroom. Running through a "to do" list, or planning the menu for the next meal, are simple examples of distractive thoughts that work well to calm the bladder. Most people have experienced being en route to the bathroom when an unexpected conversation at a party prevented it, thus ending the urge to go. Consider this technique as being one of "mind over bladder"!

Deep, cleansing, yoga-like breaths also can help. They create a relaxation response in the body, the bladder included. Breathe in deeply, exhale slowly and fully, and make your next breath in even deeper.

In the next section we give you the amazing recipe that will make the urge to urinate go away, without even using the bathroom. It worked for Emily and it will work for you, too. Use this new element of your home program to "turn off" your urge until it is time to go, according to your schedule. Try these amazing urge suppression techniques today to take charge of your waterworks!

YOUR HOME PROGRAM FOR
URGE SUPPRESSION TECHNIQUES

- Stay still by sitting or standing. *Do not move* or race to the bathroom. This will only make the bladder contract harder and make the pelvic floor muscle exercises less effective, causing leakage.
- Do six strong[1] pelvic floor muscle contractions, holding each for two seconds (see Chapter 2).
- Do *not think* about the bathroom. This defeats the purpose, because the brain is too vulnerable to the power of suggestion. Focus on something other than going to the bathroom, such as mentally creating a detailed to-do list, visualizing your favorite vacation spot, listing the items in a personal collection, or naming all of your family members' full names and birthdays. A technique that works well for golfers is to think of each hole on a golf course and its par score. Anything that requires detailed thinking and recall is good to use. A categorical topic (e.g., menu planning for your next few meals) that can be used repeatedly is ideal.
- Take *two deep breaths* with long exhalations to send a relaxation response to your overactive bladder.
- *Repeat* all of the preceding steps, if necessary, to make the urge disappear.
- You then have two choices:

  1. *Walk quietly to the bathroom.* Do not rush. Keep squeezing the pelvic floor muscles while walking slowly. Keep the mind focused on something *other* than going to the bathroom. OR
  2. *Delay* using the bathroom until it is time to go, per the voiding schedule, or until it is simply a more convenient time.

- Use the Daily Voiding Diary (see page 245) to gradually achieve a longer time between trips to the bathroom. Start with what is

---

[1] If your bladder urgency possesses the strength of Hercules, but your pelvic floor muscles are more like Gumby, then you will need to spend about four weeks strengthening your pelvic floor muscles before this will work (see Chapter 3). Your pelvic floor muscles must be strong enough for your brain to sense that you are actually contracting them, so they will win out over your bladder.

currently comfortable and *increase by half-hour increments* per week, until the normal three- to four-hour interval is achieved. This is about five to seven voids per day, with no nighttime voids.

It is very important to understand that, to cure your urge urinary incontinence, you must gain control over your bladder by retraining it. This means *not* going to the bathroom while the urge is present. Giving in to the urge only reinforces that the bladder is in charge. You should not let your bladder send you to the bathroom. You should first suppress the urge to urinate.

Next, you should go to the bathroom to void when it is more convenient for you, or when your voiding schedule says that it is time. Even if you don't think you have to go, it is very important to go at the timed interval and not skip it. Waiting for the urge to appear is counterproductive. In this way, you will experience a calm, controlled trip to the bathroom, as nature intended.

These *urge suppression techniques* give Emily the confidence to do her bladder retraining without fear of leakage. She is so thrilled to have less urgency; less frequency, resulting in fewer and fewer bathroom trips; and less urge incontinence! Knowing that she has this secret weapon against her urgency makes her feel more relaxed and confident, even when she is out of the house. Anxiety makes urgency and urge incontinence worse. Because she is calmer now, Emily feels free. In turn, her bladder is less often out of her control.

Suppress *every* urinary urge with these proven techniques and stick with your increasing schedule of urinating, progressing by thirty minutes weekly. In a few weeks, you will stop bathroom mapping during errands around your hometown and begin taking long car trips instead!

IDENTIFYING AND CORRECTING SLEEP DEPRIVATION

Sleep is one of the most effective preventative medicines we can prescribe for our own health and well-being. It is very powerful. It strengthens our immune system, repairs our muscles, and regenerates our brain to perform optimally. Unfortunately, sleep deprivation or sleep interruption stunts the progress of rebuilding that our bodies depend on during sleep.

Like Emily, people who suffer from nocturia do not receive the benefits gained through a full night's sleep. It is true that most adults should get seven to eight hours of sleep each night, and although

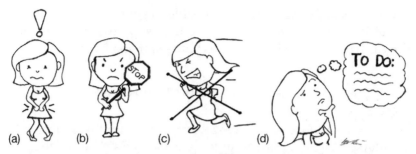

Urge suppression techniques at a glance. Panels, left to right: (a) Urge feeling! (b) Stop and be still: Do six 2-second pelvic floor contractions. (c) Do not rush to the toilet. (d) Distract yourself: Take two deep breaths; Repeat!

studies have shown that our muscles can benefit from lying in a resting state, it takes actual sleep to help supply our brains with the proper type of rest.

Different cycles of our sleep affect different parts of our brains. In adults, REM sleep typically occupies twenty percent to twenty-five percent, or 90 to 120 minutes, of each night's sleep. REM sleep is responsible for archiving our memories. It is during this stage that dreaming occurs. Without REM sleep, something we learned one day could be forgotten the next, or our recollection of an event could become foggy.

Other cycles of sleep are responsible for feeding the portions of our brains dedicated to physical health, including speech. Repetitive cycles of deep sleep (lasting about 90 minutes and alternating with REM sleep) are necessary for clear speech. This is why many sleep-deprived people have slurred speech. Others may appear groggy or confused and often function at a much slower pace than well-rested individuals. Many times, people who exhibit these symptoms are perceived as drunk, unsociable, or (as in Emily's case) showing signs of dementia.

Armed with her new training and tools, Emily gets her bladder storing urine for longer daytime periods. Then, two of the three nighttime voids disappear automatically. She is elated! However, she is still getting up once a night, and she would like to be rid of that void, too, so she tries the urge suppression techniques at night, in bed, instead of getting up to use the bathroom. Her bladder "gives in," and the urge sensation goes away as she rolls over and goes back to sleep without urinating. She finds it much easier to perform the urge suppression techniques while lying in bed, instead of walking barefoot on the cold tile floor of her bathroom, turning on the light, sitting on the cold toilet seat, washing her hands in cold water, and then being wide awake and unable to get back to sleep. Once her bladder has quieted through the urge suppression techniques, she easily returns to sleep. Try this yourself if you have nocturia.

USE YOUR URGE SUPPRESSION TECHNIQUES IN BED

Try to stay in bed by doing your urge suppression techniques instead of giving in to your bladder and urinating, thus reinforcing that *it* is in charge of *you*. Be persistent and overcome your sleep deprivation this way. Wake up in the morning full of vigor and vitality!

NOTE: Drink your last beverage two hours before bedtime or your full bladder will wake you up. (If you have medications that you take before bed, take them early.)

Within a few weeks, Emily is happily sleeping through the entire night, and so is her husband. Her bladder is not waking her and demanding to be emptied. Trips to the bathroom are a thing of the past, thanks to her successful bladder retraining. She is able to sleep the night away.

Emily is now free of the shackles put on her by her own bladder. She describes a sense of freedom that she hasn't known in years, and it shows. Uninterrupted sleep turns the formerly cranky and depressed Emily into a happy lady. She cannot remember the last time she felt this rested and energized. Emily is renewed, and she attributes this to her physical therapist and her own steadfast determination to faithfully do her home exercises and bladder retraining. Changing her behavior was easy. Her friends and family notice the obvious and profound difference in her attitude.

If you get up at night, resist your nighttime trips to the bathroom by using the urge suppression techniques, as Emily did. You will be amazed at how a good night's sleep affects every aspect of your life, improves your energy, and enhances your personality and relationships. You will feel revived, like a fresh, new woman, ready to celebrate life!

THE DIET AND HYDRATION PLAN

Many different foods and beverages can irritate the bladder. Emily used to consume some of the traditional culprits: caffeine, orange juice, alcohol, and spicy food. Her flatulence problem was largely due to dietary choices as well. Cutting back on the sugar-free and other gas-yielding foods will make a big difference. Also, she now possesses the pelvic floor strength to prevent the untimely escape of gas.

No one really knows why certain dietary choices affect the bladder the way they do. Moreover, one individual may be more susceptible to a certain food than another person. This is why using a daily log can be so powerful in making diagnoses. A food or drink that irritates an individual's bladder will cause it to contract. The contracting bladder brings on a strong need to urinate, and it compounds all of the incontinence problems that individual may face.

Emily could begin by eliminating all of the bladder-irritating foods from her diet. After a week or so, she can add a food or drink back into her diet, one at a time, and note in her daily diary any effect this has.

This does not mean she has to give up her their favorite foods or drinks entirely. She may be able to enjoy them in moderation; she should just expect to do more urge suppressing!

How much should Emily drink? Emily is underhydrated and could even be labeled dehydrated. One rule of thumb that works well is to divide Emily's 160 pounds of body weight by two, which yields the number 80. This number, in ounces, would be good daily fluid intake for Emily; that is, 80 ounces of beverages per day would be good for her body size. This formula is more specific to the individual than the general trend to simply say "eight glasses of water per day" regardless of body weight. Shaquille O'Neal would need much more fluid than Emily, and a petite, 100-pound woman would need even less fluid intake than Emily.

At first, Emily thought 80 ounces sounded like too much. Once she divided the 80 ounces over the course of her day, she realized it was only about 5.5 ounces per hour. And she made sure to keep the two hours before bedtime beverage-free.

HOW MUCH SHOULD I DRINK IN A DAY?

Take your body weight and divide this number by two. That number—in ounces—is the amount of fluid (from all types of beverages) that you should consume daily. Drink more if you are exercising heavily or talking excessively, thereby losing fluid through perspiration and water vapor; drink less if you eat juicy fruits and vegetables.

NOTE: Drink throughout the day, just not 2 hours before bedtime.

Do you drink half your body weight, in ounces? If you need to drink more, this fluid increase will not trigger more trips to the bathroom, because you are armed with your urge suppression techniques that teach your bladder to relax and store more urine, up to its 16-ounce capacity. Moreover, adding fluid will help dilute irritating acids in your bladder, yielding clearer, less concentrated urine. You should, however, space your fluid intake throughout the day so your body stays well hydrated, making the voiding schedule easier to follow.

You may drink nothing when you are out of the house and then try to "catch up" when you arrive home, feeling extremely thirsty. This bingeing and withholding of fluids aggravates an already-overactive bladder. Consistency is what will successfully retrain your bladder.

Water is always the best beverage choice, but it can be flavored with a small amount of fruit juice for more variety, if desired. Diluted orange juice or grapefruit juice will not be as irritating to the bladder as drinking these acidic juices full strength, and dilution saves calories as well. Adding fruit juice to sparkling water offers a healthy alternative to diet sodas. There are many other ways to successfully substitute with beverages that are less irritating to the bladder.

Coffee is a double whammy: It contains the acidity of citrus juices plus the caffeine of cola products. Emily will benefit if she switches either to decaffeinated coffee or to a low-acid coffee with caffeine (available at healthier food stores, e.g., Trader Joe's).

Like acidic foods and drinks, alcohol can cause the bladder to contract. In addition, because alcohol is a central nervous system depressant, it causes all of the muscles in the body to relax. The pelvic floor, a skeletal muscle, also relaxes and will weaken under the influence of alcohol. That effect creates another obstacle for an incontinent person to overcome.

Emily does enjoy an occasional glass of wine, and she should simply remain aware of its effects on her bladder problem. She doesn't want to feel deprived of her favorite foods and beverages, and her physical therapist agrees with this philosophy. Now she can choose her occasions wisely and drink wine when a bathroom is handy. Most important, she will know to blame the alcohol—and not herself—if she falls off her bladder retraining schedule because of the added urgency. In the next table we give you a handy substitution guide, which will allow you to make informed decisions on what you choose to eat and drink.

YOUR HOME PROGRAM FOR DIETARY SUBSTITUTIONS AND HYDRATION

<u>Bladder Irritant</u>	<u>Substitution</u>
Coffee	Low-acid regular coffee: ■ Available at Trader Joe's or other health food stores Decaffeinated coffee: ■ Kava (low-acid instant) ■ Postum or Pero
Tea	Noncitrus herbal teas
Orange or grapefruit juice	Low-acid fruit juices: ■ Grape ■ Apple ■ Pear ■ Apricot ■ Papaya Or dilute orange juice with water or make flavored water Take a vitamin: ■ Calcium carbonate cobuffered with calcium ascorbate Eat a low-acid fruit instead: ■ Apricots ■ Papayas ■ Watermelon ■ Pears
Artificially sweetened diet sodas	■ Mix any fruit juice with sparkling water
Alcoholic beverages	■ Concord grape juice served in a wine glass ■ Nonalcoholic wine ■ Low-alcohol beer

Hydration

Divide your body weight by two. That number, in ounces, is your guide to estimating how much you should drink per day (based on your size).

Although the foods one consumes can be identified as irritants, there are other adversaries to consider. Smoking can be extremely irritating to the bladder and the bladder wall. The nicotine found in cigarettes can cause an increase in urinary frequency and urinary urgency. Smoking also can cause coughing, which can prove detrimental to an individual with stress incontinence. The additional pressure from excessive, chronic coughing can cause the pelvic floor muscles to become fatigued, resulting in more stress incontinence.

Medications, whether natural or not, can cause an increase in bladder problems. Ask your doctor or pharmacist about the over-the-counter or prescription drugs you take.

We sincerely hope that now you are infused with the knowledge and motivation to start your bladder retraining, committed to regaining control of your bladder and your life. Here is the short version of what you learned in this rather long—but inspirational (we hope)—chapter on urge urinary incontinence. Learn to control your bladder gracefully, as nature intended.

A Quick Outline

YOUR HOME PROGRAM
FOR URGE URINARY INCONTINENCE

- **Strengthen Your Pelvic Floor:**
  Spend about four weeks building your pelvic floor strength as outlined in Chapter 3.
- **Complete a Voiding Diary:**
  Enlarge and copy the form in Appendix II, page 245. Fill it out completely for twenty-four hours. This is your first step. Follow the directions in the section titled "YOUR HOME PROGRAM: HOW TO COMPLETE A VOIDING DIARY" (p. 99).
- **Analyze Your Voiding Diary:**
  How often do you urinate, day and night? Exactly what triggers your leakage: physical activity, beverages, food, running water, or arriving home? Decide whether you have stress, urge, or mixed urinary incontinence. How many leaks are you having? How many pads are you using? Use the analysis provided in the "ANALYZING A VOIDING DIARY" section (p. 100).

■ **Retrain Your Bladder:**
Starting with your current time interval on your diary, keep broadening it by adding thirty minutes every week. Continue adding time to stretch out your bathroom visits until they are three to four hours apart. See the "YOUR HOME PROGRAM: HOW TO RETRAIN YOUR BLADDER" section (p. 105).

■ **Use Your Urge Suppression Techniques**

☐ **Daytime:** Try to suppress every urge you get during the day. After suppressing, *either* walk calmly to the bathroom (because it *is time*, per your schedule) or delay until your next scheduled trip.

☐ **Nighttime:** Try to remain in bed by doing your urge suppression techniques, instead of giving in to your bladder and reinforcing that *it* is in charge of *you*. Overcome your sleep deprivation this way! The sections titled "YOUR HOME PROGRAM FOR URGE SUPPRESSION TECHNIQUES" (p. 109) and "IDENTIFYING AND CORRECTING SLEEP DEPRIVATION" (p. 110) will teach you how.

■ **Make Dietary Substitutions:**
After identifying your known bladder irritants, be smart about ingesting them. Caffeine, alcohol, and acidic drinks are the biggest culprits. If you choose to consume them, get ready to do extra urge suppressing, and enjoy them in moderation! In the previous section we offered many easy substitutions.

■ **Stay Well Hydrated:**
Drink half your body weight—in ounces—daily. Space your intake evenly throughout your day. Drink more if you are more active or are talking an excessive amount, to offset perspiration and water vapor loss. Do not drink anything at least 2 hours before bedtime to minimize nocturia.

Take your completed Daily Voiding Diary to your next doctor's appointment and discuss your urinary incontinence with him or her. This can be your primary care doctor, your obstetrician/gynecologist, a urologist, or a urogynecologist, the one with whom you feel most comfortable talking. Rest assured, your physician will view your incontinence merely as the medical condition that it is, without passing judgment. Impress your doctor with your knowledge and the accurate history of your problem contained in your voiding diary! Use Appendix III, page 247, to find a physical therapist in your area who specializes in Women's Health, or ask your doctor to help you locate one. You will be a "star" patient if you come to your first visit armed with all of this knowledge!

Urge incontinence is treatable and curable with behavioral modifications, so there is no reason to suffer with it. A study of 197 women, published in the *Journal of the American Medical Association*, found bladder retraining to be more effective and more acceptable to the study participants than drug treatment (Burgio et al., 1998). The authors concluded that "Behavioral treatment is a safe and effective conservative intervention that should be made more readily available to patients as a first-line treatment for urge and mixed incontinence" (Burgio et al., 1998, p. 1995). Furthermore, there are no side effects and no risks with this approach!

Physical therapy is accepted mainstream medicine and is covered by Medicare and most insurance plans. Why wait another day? Don't endure it, cure it!

> "When the student is ready, the master appears."
> —Buddhist proverb

6 Your Treatment Plan: Adding Pilates

"HARD CORE": MEET KIM PERELLI, COAUTHOR

*T*he birth of my first child was one of the most memorable moments of my life. Little did I know at the time, however, that the process of having her would cause such great bodily harm! Okay, well, that's a slight exaggeration, and she was well worth it—but let's just say, things have never been the same again. The piles of "mommy-to-be" books I consumed during my pregnancy prepared me for the sleepless nights and the many different challenges that accompany a newborn. But what no one ever told me was that I could become incontinent.

I became aware of my problem just six weeks after my daughter was born. I entered the gym for the first time and decided to go for an easy run on the treadmill. As I began to pick up the pace, I suddenly realized I was wetting my pants. Soon I was soaked! Grateful for my tattered dark blue running pants, I tied my sweatshirt around my waist, slowly dismounted the treadmill, and hobbled out of the gym like a cowboy from a spaghetti western.

Horrified at this experience, I shared it with my OB/GYN, who assured me this was "all very typical" and advised me to wait until I was "finished having kids" before I addressed any sort of fix. So I took her advice and decided to wait.

After my sweet boy came into the world twenty-two months later, I was determined to run again. My incontinence affected my life in no other way, and I missed running tremendously.

My OB/GYN referred me to a renowned female urologist, who recommended urodynamic testing that would detect any anatomical problems with my bladder, kidneys, urinary tract, etc. The night before my urology appointment, I realized an enema was needed prior to my visit, and the procedure itself would involve catheters! Not at all pleased, but desperate to get help, I forged ahead.

Upon my arrival, I was told to use the bathroom. The medical techni-cian motioned toward an odd-looking chair in the middle of the examination room. The chair was the toilet, and it was connected to an adjacent com-puter with wires. After I went on my own, my bladder was then drained some more via catheter. An additional catheter was placed in the only other opening available—yes, in my rectum—and surface electrodes were placed on my bottom to record pelvic floor activity. "Are we having fun yet?"

Next, my catheterized bladder was refilled with water. My ability to hold liquid was monitored and recorded under stress-inducing situations like coughing and laughing, and my pelvic floor activity was recorded. The feeling was reminiscent of standing at the end of a long line during half-time at a Trojan football game. Worse yet, the technician kept suggesting over and over, "Do you have to go yet?" Gritting my teeth, I held on as long as I could with (what felt like) a gallon of water floating around in my bladder.

In the end, the test proved futile. I had no leakage during the test, and no clear anatomical problems were identified. Once again I was diag-nosed with stress urinary incontinence, based on what had happened at the gym—something I knew before the appointment. And while the urologist could have performed further testing, the enema, the double catheteriza-tion, and the prophylactic antibiotic given afterward were enough for me; instead I chose to seek the other avenue she suggested: physical therapy.

About a week later, I entered the physical therapy clinic, bracing myself for whatever waited on the other side of the door. In the physical therapist's waiting room, however, unlike the one in the urology office, I wasn't the only younger patient. Here, there was a feeling of hope and rehabilitation! My first appointment with physical therapist Kathryn Kassai, was downright delightful! Kathryn was peppy and positive and had the bedside manner of your favorite childhood teacher, who immediately put you at ease with her soothing demeanor. There were no instruments inserted into me, no shock treatment, and no post-appointment pills to pop. It was all very natural.

My weekly physical therapy sessions combined surface electromyo-graph biofeedback with my home program. I got so skilled with the biofeed-back that I once joked that I could write my name on the graph using my pelvic floor muscles! Soon I was running again, leak-free! It was incredibly simple. I will be forever grateful to the urologist who sent me to physical therapy.

Midway through my treatment, I was introduced to the Pilates Reformer exercise approach. I was taught how to engage my pelvic floor muscles dur-ing a Pilates workout and concentrate on building my core strength.

Today, I continue to do my daily exercises and participate in Pilates Reformer classes as part of my maintenance program. Not only has Pilates helped my incontinence issues, it has given me incredible core strength, better balance, and improved posture. Both my life and my body have been transformed.

My own experience with urinary incontinence was clearly good research for this book; however, it was the millions of women I learned about—the ones who suffer in silence—who prompted me to share my story. Finally, the realization that women of sound mind (despite weak pelvic floors) are being placed in nursing homes prematurely is what broke my heart. My big problem was that I couldn't run, but there were so many more women out there who couldn't live—*or at least not live the full and rich lives they deserved. Hence,* The Bathroom Key *was born.*

Pregnancy and childbirth are leading causes of stress urinary incontinence among women. Like Kim, many mothers experience their initial episode of incontinence either during pregnancy or after delivery. Some women have only a slight problem, which goes away a few weeks after delivery; others, however, experience incontinence with any sort of impact to their bodies. In Kim's case, it was running. For many others incontinence can be triggered just by stepping off a curb or by one of the most typical causes, such as sneezing, coughing, or laughing. Sadly, many new mothers just accept their newly acquired condition as a consequence of having a baby. We have heard so many women say, "Oh, everyone has it— it's just part of having a baby," or "Just wear a pad. It's no big deal." These women wear pads all month long and carry their own extra underwear in their baby's diaper bag. This is very sad and totally unnecessary.

> Unfortunately, the advice that Kim received from her OB/ GYN—about waiting until she was finished having kids to do anything about her incontinence—was bad advice. Women can get physical therapy or do the pelvic floor strengthening exercises in a home program before, during, and in between pregnancies. The more training the pelvic floor gets, the stronger it becomes, no matter when.

Some advertising moguls would like us to believe there are only three options for controlling incontinence: (a) pads, (b) pharmaceuticals, or (c) surgery. We are here to tell you there is *one more option—* the *right* one—that should be tried first. It is natural, noninvasive, and, as Kim remarked, "simple." For those of you who have experienced relief from physical therapy and/or from the techniques you have learned in your home program as presented so far in this book, get ready: We have something wonderful to add.

JOSEPH PILATES AND THE CORE MUSCLES

Long before the likes of Arnold Schwarzenegger lumbered onto the fitness scene, and decades before the jumpsuit-clad Jack LaLanne flexed his biceps, there was a man who many believe was the true guru of fitness. His name was Joseph Hubertus Pilates. As with Dr. Arnold Kegel, the Pilates name has become synonymous with

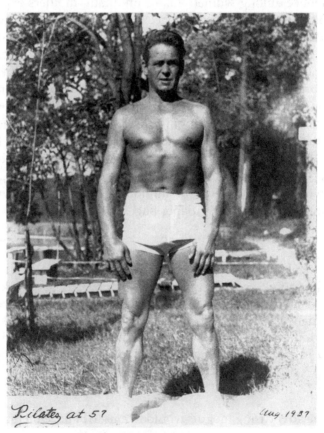

Pilates at 57   *Aug. 1937*

Joseph H. Pilates, age 57, in 1937.
Used with permission of Sean Gallagher, PT.

his life mission. In the case of Pilates, his life mission was ultimate health. He believed in the powerful relationship among mind, body, and spirit.

Born in Germany in 1880, Pilates was a visionary. He phrased it best himself when he said, "My work is 50 years ahead of its time," and it was. As a child, Pilates was sickly, suffering from rickets, asthma, and rheumatic fever. A skinny kid, he was often bullied, and he even lost an eye, presumably during one incessant attack. This childhood taunting was thought to be the catalyst for his career quest to become physically and mentally strong. He began to study self-defense and became obsessed with the composition of the human body.

Pilates's philosophies may not have strayed too far from his family tree. His father was described as a champion gymnast and gym manager. His mother practiced naturopathic principles, believing that the body could heal itself. His parents' backgrounds are most likely the sources for his own early beliefs. As a youngster, Pilates began studying anatomy books and soon memorized every muscle in the body. He studied both Eastern and Western exercise interpretations, including yoga, zen, and ancient practices from the Greeks and Romans. By age fourteen, he was so physically well developed he was used as a male model for anatomy charts.

A well-rounded athlete, Pilates found success as a boxer, gymnast, skier, and diver. After moving to England, he worked for years in a circus act. Because he was a native German, during World War I he was placed in various internment camps for so called "enemy aliens." At the camps, he developed a uniquely effective form of exercise, which he called *Contrology*. The name *Pilates*, referring to the exercise philosophy, came much later.

At some camps, Pilates taught wrestling and self-defense to the other German nationals. Later, he was stationed in the infirmary with many bedridden and weak German soldiers. Using cast-off bedsprings, Pilates fashioned pieces of resistance equipment and made all of the bedridden soldiers participate in his exercise regimen. He realized that adding the resistive coils forced the body's deeper muscles to work.

During that time, a flu epidemic spread throughout the world, killing millions. The internment camp was also plagued, and many people died. However, not one of Pilates's students perished from the flu. Pilates believed his fellow comrades' immune systems would become stronger after exercising—and indeed they did. His contraption was the first of its kind, and it was probably the first crude prototype of today's Pilates Reformer machines.

After the war, and at the urging of family living in the United States, Pilates moved to America. On the ship to New York City he met Clara, the woman who would soon become his wife. Joe and Clara opened a gym on Eighth Avenue in Manhattan, in a building that housed many dance studios. During that period, he enhanced the methods of *Contrology*. He believed emphatically that muscle strength and flexibility could be gained by efficient breathing and controlled slow movement that focused directly on the muscle itself. He created a program that joined mental focus, body movement, and smooth breathing to help rehabilitate while increasing strength, flexibility, balance, and posture. Pilates did not believe it was possible to get the same muscle development from a fast-paced cardiovascular workout. Modern-day physiology supports this.

Using bench-like tables in his gym, Pilates hooked resistance cables to them so his students could attach their hands and feet during exercise. The photo on the next page shows Joe, Clara, and

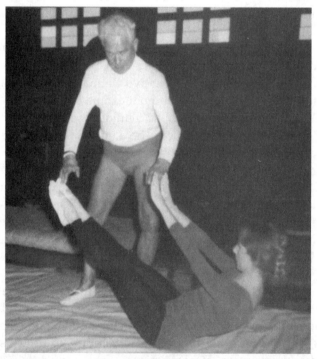

Joseph Pilates instructing student Romana Kryzanowska in the early 1960s. Used with permission of Sean Gallagher, PT.

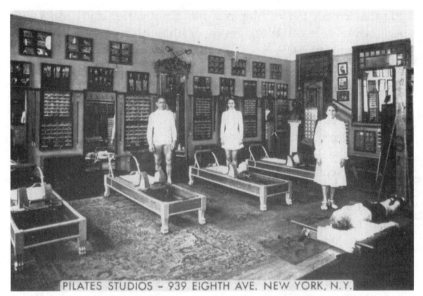

PILATES STUDIOS - 939 EIGHTH AVE. NEW YORK, N.Y.

Joseph H. Pilates (left) and Clara Pilates (far right) in their first New York City studio (located in their apartment), circa 1920s. The original claw-feet Reformers are shown.
Used with permission of Sean Gallagher, PT.

claw-footed Reformers in their first New York City studio. Notice the serial photographs on the wall: Pilates felt compelled to document and preserve his unique exercises for posterity. We are ever so glad he did!

Joe began to work with many of the dancers in his building, helping them to rehabilitate after injuries and showing them how to gain core muscle strength to prevent future injuries. He created a spectrum of exercises to isolate muscles and make them work from the inside out, using the resistance springs he added to his machines. All of his exercises were designed to be performed in a sitting, kneeling, or lying-down position. He believed this was less stressful to the heart, lungs, and bladder, allowing flowing and natural movement. He believed in slow, controlled repetition. If a student could do only a few repetitions of an exercise, Pilates would stop that student until he or she could build enough stamina to correctly complete the full set of repetitions. He would not allow *form* to suffer. He felt that five perfect repetitions were more effective than 100 fast or sloppy ones. He believed in "the attainment and maintenance of a uniformly developed body with a sound mind fully capable of naturally, easily, and satisfactorily performing our many and varied daily tasks with spontaneous zest and pleasure—everything should be smooth, like a cat" (Thomson, 2003).

Pilates lived to age eighty-six. He had a *huge* presence and an often authoritative manner. He was lovingly referred to as a "lion" in his obituary (*New York Times, October 10, 1967*); however, he was also a caring soul with a very altruistic side that may have stemmed from his own childhood adversities. He spread his message generously in the hope that those he touched would benefit from his wisdom. He can help you, too. The following famous quote of his invites you to embark upon your own Pilates journey: "In ten sessions you'll FEEL a difference, in twenty you'll SEE a difference, and in thirty sessions, you'll have a whole new body."

Cheers, Joe. Danke schön!

THE MANY BENEFITS OF PILATES

The exercise approach that Joseph Pilates developed nearly 100 years ago still has widespread application today. The name *Contrology* never caught on; instead, it was Pilates's own surname that has stood the test of time. In 2005, there were 11 million Americans practicing Pilates regularly, and the number continues to grow (Ellin, 2005). Pilates is embraced by a broad cross-section of the population and offers multigenerational appeal. One of the finest features of a Pilates workout is its inherent ease on the body. Unlike many other exercise programs, Pilates exercises are low-impact ones that do not cause undue stress to the tendons, ligaments, muscles, and bones. On the contrary, Pilates is designed to support the joints and lengthen muscles, making them stronger and more limber. Through targeted exercise of the internal muscles, more flexibility and fluid mobility result. Thus, Pilates exercise can be enjoyed by teenagers and seniors alike. Athletes, fitness trainers, Pilates instructors, and physical therapists are convinced that the principles are sound and the benefits bountiful.

In 1992, physical therapist Sean Gallagher purchased the Pilates trademark. The purchase encompassed Joseph Pilates's entire collection of photographs and blueprint designs, as well as his original equipment. Gallagher is credited with copyrighting and printing the first Pilates training manual, with the goal of spreading the Pilates method within the physical therapy community and beyond. With

Pilates's photographs in his possession, Gallagher was able to remain authentic to the proper Pilates techniques. This collection of archived photographs depicts Pilates himself modeling the precise angle and position of each step of each exercise. Recognizing the infinite benefits the Pilates approach could bring to physical therapy, Gallagher shared this historical treasure with the world in his book, *The Joseph H. Pilates Archive Collection: Photographs, Writings, and Designs* (Gallagher & Kryzanowska, 2000).

In homage to the master himself, Pilates exercise is taught with precision in physical therapy clinics and exercise studios around the globe; however, no two Pilates classes are alike. There are so many exercises that your body gets what it needs: variety! Forget about distracting yourself by watching TV as you pedal mindlessly on a stationary bike. Pilates requires focus, control, and coordination. Although strength is definitely needed as well, you can begin at any level and advance as you gain more power. The main requirement is a willingness on your part to concentrate on your movement. The mind–body connection was a primary tenet for Joseph Pilates, just as it was for Dr. Arnold Kegel.

As we share, in the sections that follow, the enormous benefits of a Pilates workout with you, we want you first to understand the unique aspects of the exercise. To begin with, much of a Pilates workout is done lying down. Unlike circuit training at a gym, in Pilates there is one piece of equipment that serves as the staple for the entire workout: the Pilates Reformer.

The Pilates Reformer

Pilates's most successful and popular invention clearly is the Pilates Reformer. Modern reformers are eight feet long and resemble a low, narrow bench (about one and a half feet off the floor). No electricity is required, because the sliding carriage is powered by human effort—namely, the arms, legs, and core.

Many Reformers have sheepskin-covered stirrups (often referred to as the "large fuzzies") for the feet and smaller sheepskin-covered handles ("small fuzzies") for the hands. Either the hands or feet are in the fuzzies at a particular time. The fuzzies are connected to cables as part of a pulley system. Movement of the padded carriage occurs when one pulls on the fuzzies or pushes off from the stationary foot bar.

Resistance comes from four or five springs or cords. Each exercise can be done with more or less resistance by varying the number of springs/cords in use according to the individual's ability level. Surprisingly, *less* resistance makes some exercises *harder*! You'll see examples of this later in this chapter.

An adjustable headrest allows proper positioning of the head and neck. The foot bar can be removed and replaced with an ancillary piece of equipment called a *Jump Board*, which provides more aerobic conditioning in conjunction with a very tough core workout.

Exercises on the Pilates Reformer can be performed while one is lying, kneeling, sitting, standing, or lying on one's side. With over 500 different exercises, the Pilates Reformer is the most versatile piece of exercise equipment ever invented. And to think it was designed nearly 100 years ago! There are many models of quality Pilates Reformers for home or clinic use; one example is shown below. Contact information and discount pricing are offered in Appendix IV, page 252.

A one-hour Pilates session (which can include 30 or more different exercises) is equivalent to many hours at a traditional gym. Pilates represents the epitome of total-body conditioning, with the core muscles of the *pelvic brace* at its foundation. You can expect many benefits from the Pilates approach. The incredible thing is that you get *all* of the benefits in one exercise session.

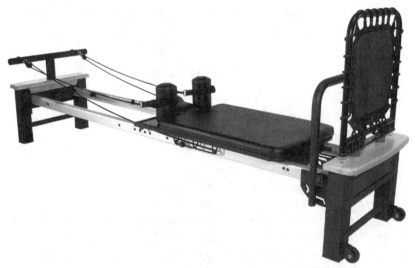

The AeroPilates® ProXP556 Pilates Reformer, by Stamina® Products, Inc, with the Jump Board in place.
Used with permission from Stamina Products.

Strengthening and Toning of the Core Muscles

Naturally the core muscles include the pelvic brace muscles (the pelvic floor and the transversus abdominus). Other core muscles that Pilates targets are the buttocks; the inner thighs; and the deep paraspinal muscles (thick muscles located on each side of the spine). The accessory muscle exercise you learned in Chapter 3 is really a pre-Pilates exercise that targets these same core muscles isometrically. Reformer exercises begin on your back, but they quickly progress into the sitting, kneeling, standing, side-lying, and lying-on-your-tummy (prone) positions.

Patients who need rehabilitation can benefit from Pilates. Because Pilates includes exercises performed in the recumbent position (lying on the back), gentle resistive exercises can be added to therapeutic exercise programs at an earlier stage. For example, resisted squats can be done on the Reformer without one's full body weight causing too much strain on a postoperative knee joint. A patient with lower back pain can begin strengthening his back sooner (without making his pain worse), because the carriage of the Reformer supports his back and Pilates exercises do not require that he move it. Strengthening the core muscles that stabilize the back is a pain-free way to start the rehabilitation process. Elderly individuals often are delighted that so much valuable exercise can take place while they lie on their backs!

Professional and nonprofessional athletes have embraced Pilates to enhance their athletic performance. A baseball will fly farther if the batter has strong deep abdominal muscles. A field goal kicker will send the ball farther if his core is engaged at the time of the kick. A tennis player will deliver a stronger serve if her pelvic brace stabilizes her trunk, so that the power of her swing can transfer to the ball instead of back into her trunk.

Reduction of Incontinence

In Chapter 3 we taught you how everyday activities can put internal resistance on your pelvic floor and the deep abdominal muscles. Taking this concept to the next level, Pilates Reformer and mat exercises give you a systematic way to put resistance on your pelvic brace muscles, thereby further reducing your stress incontinence and making your urge suppression techniques more effectual. The stronger your pelvic floor is, the quicker you will win the war over your bladder. Pilates exercises are used by physical therapists who specialize in Women's Health issues for this very reason.

Improved Posture

Some muscles are designed for motion; others (e.g., the core muscles of the pelvic floor and the transversus abdominus) are designed for static postural support of your organs and of your spine. The stronger these muscles are, the better your posture will be. Countless professional dancers have superb posture due to years of training with Pilates. Indeed, some dancers are the best Pilates instructors! Physical therapists use a Pilates-based therapeutic exercise plan to improve slouched postures in patients of all ages.

Pilates will give you a flatter tummy along with taller posture. As you learned in Chapter 3, Pilates targets the transversus abdominus, and resistance strengthens it. Sit-ups are not aimed at the deep transversus abdominus. Sit-ups selectively strengthen the superficial "six-pack" (rectus abdominus) muscle that has very little to do with posture or flat abs.

Improved Balance

Did you try the standing-on-one-leg balancing exercise in Chapter 3? Remember how contracting your transversus abdominus kept your hips level, even as you raised one leg off the floor? Well, Pilates exercises put actual resistance on your transversus abdominus to make your balance even more outstanding. Physical therapists and athletic trainers incorporate Pilates balance activities that recruit the core in order to improve walking after hip surgery or ankle sprains.

Improved Coordination

An average Pilates class comprises thirty or more exercises. Many are done in combination with each other. Think of it as dancing on your back! This builds coordination, a benefit sorely lacking in the heavy, mindless repetitions performed on machines at most gyms. Coordination exercises foster faster reaction time by speeding up the transmission of nerve impulses. Every athlete and fitness-minded person wants better coordination, be they basketball players, gymnasts, or lacrosse players. Daily living takes plenty of coordination, and without continued challenge, physical coordination diminishes with age.

Improved Proprioception

Proprioception is defined as knowing how your body is moving without looking at it; it is your body's ability to sense where your arms and legs are positioned by "listening" to little sensors in your joints, called *Golgi tendon organs*, that transmit sensory information from your muscle tendons to your brain so you can perform coordinated movement. You don't close your eyes in a Pilates exercise, but as you lie on your back you may not be able to *see* what your legs are doing! This gives the nondancer some training in proprioception; the command "Don't look down at your feet" is common in ballroom dancing lessons. Every physical therapist wants to improve proprioception in elderly individuals, because it helps prevent falls. Stellar proprioception also improves accuracy in sports such as soccer, bowling, and the martial arts.

Improved Flexibility

In Pilates there is a strong focus on elongating the muscles. This may be partially due to Pilates's decades of work with dancers who needed extraordinarily supple muscles. All people—be they athletes, rehabilitation patients, or people with computer jobs—need stretching. Our muscles get tight and short depending on the lives we lead. No one has perfect flexibility throughout his or her entire body. It is not unusual for one person in a Pilates class to experience tightness during one exercise and for another class member to experience that same tightness during a different exercise. Strange as it may seem, most individual Pilates exercises actually stretch and strengthen at the same time! We offer you a few examples of this later in this chapter. Good form, holding certain positions, and elongating the spine and limbs are all emphasized in Pilates.

Improved Mental Alertness and Memory

What gives a person more mental alertness in his or her advancing years: crossword puzzles or exercise? Studies show that exercise does! What gives you the most improvement in mental alertness is *new* exercise, *new* movements you have never done before. In a typical Pilates session, you are bound to learn two or three entirely new exercises (because there is so much variety), and that builds new "muscle memory" in your muscle and new connections in your brain. This benefit is why people frequently feel refreshed and invigorated after a Pilates session. Most people haven't learned a new movement pattern or taken up a new sport in years. As we age, we should embrace every natural remedy to ward off memory lapse and dementia.

Reduced Stress on the Body

What Pilates does *not* do is provide heavy impact; instead, it exerts very low stress on the joints. There are few repetitions; no quick, jerky motions; no heavy weights; and no strain to the point of exhaustion. These are all good things. Many people need to adjust their expectations when they are coming from a typical gym workout perspective. The Reformer provides low resistance, but you need the core muscles of the pelvic brace to help execute the movement. The intent is for the entire body to work as a unit, instead of just one muscle working to the point of fatigue. Pilates focuses on proper breathing so that oxygen can reach all parts of the body, fostering relaxation and stress reduction.

Improved Mood

Exercise combats depression thanks to the "feel good" endorphins that the body releases. Many Pilates students participate in classes of five to fifty persons, building nice camaraderie with others, which also fights depression.

Pilates himself summarized the benefits of his approach:

> [It] is designed to give you suppleness, natural grace, and skill that will be unmistakably reflected in the way you play, and in the way you work. You will develop muscular power with corresponding endurance, ability to perform arduous duties, to play strenuous games, to walk, run, or travel for long distances without undue body fatigue or mental strain. (Gallagher and Kryzanowska, 1999)

Isn't this exactly what you'd like to have in your own life? Pilates is a great way to get there. Celebrities and professional athletes use Pilates, because their livelihood depends on looking good and being fit. The short list includes Julia Roberts, Madonna, Sharon Stone, Cameron Diaz, Sandra Bullock, NBA players, NFL players, and the New York City Ballet. Now you know the secret to their flat abs and long, lean, strong bodies.

WHO CAN DO PILATES?

- People suffering from stress and/or urge incontinence
- Professional/nonprofessional athletes from any sport
- Elderly individuals
- Teenagers
- Business professionals
- Fine arts performers and dancers
- People who suffer from chronic pain and/or joint stress
- Pregnant women (both prenatal and postpartum)
- People who suffer from stress
- People with back pain
- Overweight people

Pilates may be the remedy to cure what ails you, but you should consult a physician before beginning any new exercise regimen, especially if you are in the last trimester of pregnancy or have had any of the following health issues:

- High blood pressure
- Heart issues or heart attack
- Family history of stroke
- Frequent dizzy spells
- Extreme breathlessness after mild exertion
- Arthritis or other bone problems
- Back problems
- Severe muscular, ligament, or tendon problems
- Other known (or suspected) diseases or medical conditions

Many new students of Pilates notice a dramatic difference after their first one-hour session. The recurrent comment most women make is, "I feel taller!" This is due to the immediate postural effect resulting from enhanced core activation.

Some descriptions you may hear of the muscles targeted in Pilates exercises include the *Pilates powerhouse*, the *Pilates core*, and the *pelvic brace*. The list of individual muscles consists of the transversus abdominus, the pelvic floor, the adductors of the inner thighs, the gluteals, the deep spinal muscles, and the other abdominal muscles. Most Pilates exercises work all these muscle groups simultaneously and in natural harmony.

Pilates combines perfectly with other exercise regimens, such as spinning, swimming, water aerobics, weight lifting, running, and sport-specific exercise. It does not have to replace any form of exercise you are already doing; instead, it will be the perfect complement.

In the past decade, Pilates has exploded in popularity. *The Philadelphia Inquirer Magazine* called Pilates "the perfect exercise regimen for our time"; *The Washington Post* stated that "Pilates has quietly survived all the various fitness trends"; and the *Atlanta Journal-Constitution* claimed that "Pilates unquestionably gives results" (Gallagher & Kryzanowska, 1999, p. 1). Joseph Pilates was a genius and years ahead of his time!

How do you get started with Pilates, so you can augment your home program to overcome your incontinence? You should consult a certified Pilates instructor or physical therapist first, to ensure that you'll be using a correct and safe technique. Resources to locate one of these professionals in your area are provided in Appendix III, page 247. Many physical therapy clinics and Pilates studios offer a free or reduced-rate first session as a trial.

Once you are proficient in Pilates, there are many ways to safely perform the exercises at home (with minimal equipment or with a home version of the Reformer). Mat exercises require nothing more than a yoga mat on your living room floor. In the next two sections of this chapter, we present two versions of the Pilates approach: (a) Reformer and (b) mat exercises. With so many wonderful benefits, you really have nothing to lose—except your incontinence. Get ready for a serious core work out and bid your incontinence "Farewell!"

LEARNING REFORMER PILATES EXERCISES

The Pilates Reformer is the crown jewel in Joseph Pilates's equipment collection and the device on which he usually started his students. No other apparatus that targets the core can match its incredible benefits and versatility. With the support of the Reformer, a student can easily learn to identify and fire the innermost muscles while practicing measured breathing. The fuzzies help stabilize the trunk during exercise. Most people think that using resistive equipment makes an exercise harder, and indeed that is often the case; however, most exercises done on the Pilates Reformer become *easier* over time, thanks to the balanced support it offers. Both the Reformer and the mat programs are beneficial, but the Reformer exercises are the gold standard by which to learn about the marvelous benefits of Pilates.

As you learned earlier, and as you will see from the photographs in this chapter, the Reformer is a pulley-based system. This is advantageous because you will strengthen your arms and legs in many different planes of motion. Whereas a weight machine at the gym locks you into one plane, the Reformer allows movement in all directions—replicating how we move in life.

You can add Pilates Reformer exercises into your home program at any time. There is just one caveat to this: The earlier you start them, the more leakage you could have. These exercises will tax your deep abdominals and pelvic floor muscles (pelvic brace), and it is wise to develop some core strength first. For this reason, most physical therapists do not add Reformer exercises to an in-clinic program until the fourth or fifth week.

In addition to the Reformer itself, Pilates used various ancillary pieces of equipment to boost a Reformer workout. These include the Pilates Box, the Pilates Pole, and the Jump Board.

Pilates Box

The Pilates Box is usually used only during a Reformer Pilates session. The typical Pilates Box is sixteen inches wide, thirty inches long, and twelve inches high. The box can be placed on the Reformer in either parallel or perpendicular positions. You can sit on it or lie prone (on your belly). Adding the box improves the balance and stabilization requirements of the exercises. The box is a perfect tool that targets the trunk and upper body.

Pilates Pole

Often used in combination with the Pilates Box, the Pilates Pole is usually found in Reformer classes only. The typical pole is extendable and is used to help achieve better balance, because it functions like a supportive cane during standing work. It can also be threaded through the fuzzy handles on the Reformer, creating a rowing bar, during arm and upper body workouts.

Jump Board

The Jump Board can replace the foot bar at the end of the Reformer. The Jump Board is the one mechanism in Pilates that adds a cardio flavor to the workout. The Jump Board has a metal frame with a pliable nylon mesh interior, similar to that of a trampoline. While lying on your back, you can bounce lightly against the Jump Board, using your core strength to move the carriage back and forth. Your leg positions change throughout the routine. However, Jump Board exercises are much more about the core muscles than the legs themselves. For this reason, the resistance is kept low.

WHEN CAN I BEGIN PILATES?

It is wise to achieve some core strengthening of your pelvic brace for a few weeks before beginning Pilates; otherwise, additional leakage may occur while you exercise on the Reformer or the mat. Depending on the severity of your incontinence, four or five weeks into your home program would be a good time to add Pilates.

All of the tools just described, along with home Reformer units, are available for purchase, although it is highly recommended that you become proficient in the exercises first. If done improperly, the exercises can cause injury. For this reason, most women attend at least a dozen classes (or more) before purchasing a Pilates Reformer. Some women prefer the keen eye of an instructor or the fellowship that a class may bring. However, if you would like to have your own machine, that is great! You can duplicate your class exercises at home. Discount ordering information for home Reformers and small Pilates exercise equipment is provided in the Appendix IV, page 252.

In the sections that follow, we give you a sample of some common beginning Pilates Reformer exercises.

Leg Lower Exercise

In the photo opposite, Kim is demonstrating the Leg Lower exercise. You will notice that her feet are in the fuzzy stirrups. Can you see that the pulleys are holding and supporting her legs, with the guidance of her instructor? The resistance is *low*, resulting in gentle support, so Kim has to use her core muscles to help support her legs; however, the Reformer's partial support of the legs allows the abdominals to work a bit less, making it easier for a beginner to maintain proper form.

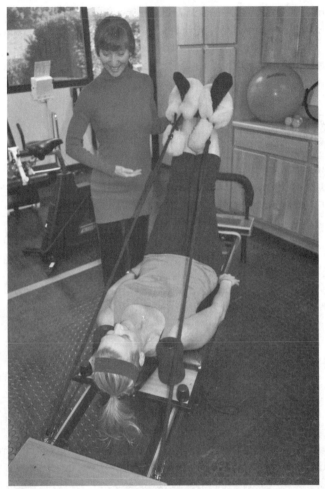

Kim performing the "Leg Lower" exercise on a Pilates Reformer, with Pilates Instructor Valyn Carenza-Pack.

Can you imagine Kim doing this same exercise *without* the support from these pulleys? If this same exercise was done on a mat, it would definitely be harder on her abdominals and pelvic floor muscles (the pelvic brace). The Leg Lower exercise can also be performed on the floor (see next section).

Directions for the Leg Lower Exercise on a Reformer:

- Place your feet in the large fuzzy stirrups.
- Position yourself as in the photo above.
- Bring your navel to your spine and squeeze your pelvic floor (the pelvic brace) and *hold*.

- Squeeze your heels together, keeping your toes apart.
- Slowly and smoothly move both legs up and down, as a unit.
- *Do not* allow *any* movement whatsoever in your trunk or back. Don't let it arch. Don't let it flatten. If your lower back arches or flattens, shorten the range so that your back stays still. Use your pelvic brace to disallow movement of your trunk.
- Repeat 10 times.
- Remember to keep breathing throughout the exercise.

Many of the 500 exercises that Pilates devised can be done recumbent, or lying on your back. This allows the outer muscles of the trunk to fully relax as you learn to work the deeper core muscles. This position also puts less strain on the bladder, heart, and other organs. It's a great starting position for elderly individuals, or for people recovering from leg injuries who are allowed only partial weight-bearing.

We now teach you a few other common Pilates Reformer exercises that are great pelvic brace strengtheners, which in turn will help you overcome your urinary incontinence faster. Exercising with a Pilates Reformer is an optional addition to your home program, but a wonderful one.

PURCHASING HOME REFORMERS

The purchase and use of home Pilates Reformers are recommended *in addition* to taking a class or receiving private instruction from a qualified Pilates instructor. Like yoga, the Pilates approach demands good form and good instruction. Without both, you increase the risk of injuring yourself. (See Appendix IV, page 252 for discount pricing.)

Advanced Leg Lower Exercise

Most Pilates exercises have several difficulty levels. If you take a Pilates class, you will see various levels of the same exercise being performed simultaneously, according to the skill levels of the individual students. Keeping the exercises challenging, yet tailored to the individual student, is the job of the Pilates instructor.

An example of an advanced version of the Leg Lower exercise is shown here. By having the head and arms work reciprocally against

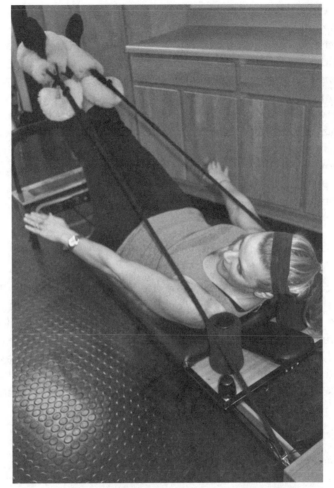

The Advanced Leg Lower exercise on a Pilates Reformer.

the legs, a more advanced exercise is created. This advanced version requires more core strength and more coordination.

Directions for the Advanced Leg Lower Exercise on a Reformer:

■ Place your feet in the large fuzzy stirrups.
■ Bring your navel to your spine and squeeze your pelvic floor (the pelvic brace) and *hold*.
■ Position your legs as pictured in above, with your legs at a 45-degree angle. Squeeze your heels together, but keep your toes apart.

- Stretch your arms long. Feel your shoulder blade muscles engage.
- Raise your head by tucking in your chin, as if to hold a lemon under your chin.
- Raise your arms as you lower your legs. As you lower your arms, raise your legs.
- *Do not* allow *any* movement whatsoever in your trunk or lower back. Don't let it arch. Don't let it flatten. If your lower back arches or flattens, squeeze your pelvic brace harder to disallow movement of your trunk or shorten the range of motion.
- Repeat 10 times.
- Remember to keep breathing throughout the exercise.

Hundred Exercise

Here, Kim is pictured performing the Hundred exercise on the Reformer. This is a foundation exercise for nearly every class Joseph Pilates taught. He felt it really helped get the circulation flowing. The Hundred rhythmically stabilizes the deep back muscles along with the pelvic brace. We will teach you how to do this exercise without a Reformer, on a mat, in the next section. As with all Pilates exercises, the goal is to hold the pelvis and trunk perfectly *still*, despite the arm and leg movements.

Directions for the Hundred Exercise on a Reformer:

- Place your hands into the small fuzzy handles.
- Bring your navel to your spine and squeeze your pelvic floor (the pelvic brace) and *hold*.
- Position your legs as pictured opposite—this is called the *tabletop leg position*—with your hips and knees at 90 degrees and your shins parallel to the floor.
- Stretch your arms alongside your body, pressing into the fuzzy handles.
- Pump your hands up and down in small (six-inch) rapid flutters. Keep your elbows straight, and your hands relaxed, and strive to make the movement come from your shoulders and shoulder blades.
- Breathe *in* for five little arm flutters and breathe *out* for five little arm flutters.
- *Do not* allow *any* movement whatsoever in your trunk or back. Don't let it arch. Don't let it flatten. If your back arches or flattens,

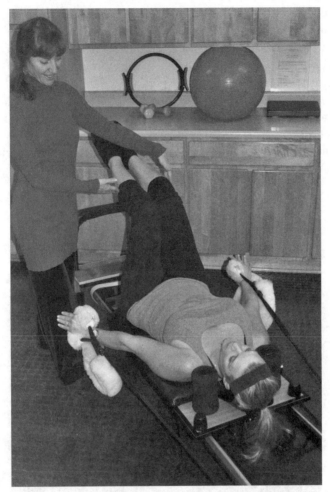

The Hundred exercise on a Pilates Reformer.

squeeze your pelvic brace harder to disallow movement of your trunk.
■ Repeat for 10 breaths, and you will have performed 100 little arm flutters.

Frog Exercise

This next Reformer exercise also can be done as a mat exercise (see next section). It adds resistance to the same muscles that are used in the accessory muscle exercise you learned in Chapter 3: the buttocks, inner thighs, pelvic floor, and transversus abdominus. On the Reformer, however, there is movement occurring, as the carriage glides back and forth with the legs moving in and out.

Directions for the Frog Exercise on a Reformer:

- Place your feet into the large fuzzy stirrups. Place your heels together, toes apart.
- Bring your navel to your spine and squeeze your pelvic floor (the pelvic brace) and *hold*.

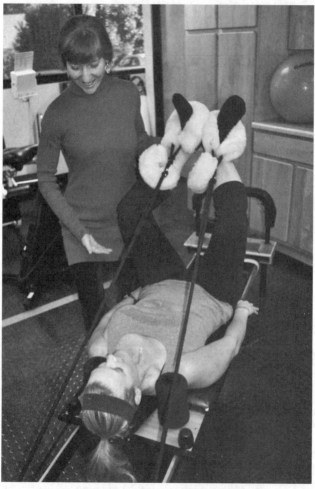

The Frog exercise on a Pilates Reformer.

- Bend your knees toward the chest as shown above.
- Straighten your knees, toward the ceiling, to a 45-degree angle.
- Bend your knees again, striving to keep the legs moving smoothly on one plane, not wavering up and down.
- *Do not* allow *any* movement whatsoever in your trunk or back. Don't let it arch. Don't let it flatten. If your back arches or flattens, shorten the motion and squeeze your pelvic brace harder to disallow movement of your trunk.
- Repeat 10 times.
- Remember to keep breathing throughout the exercise.

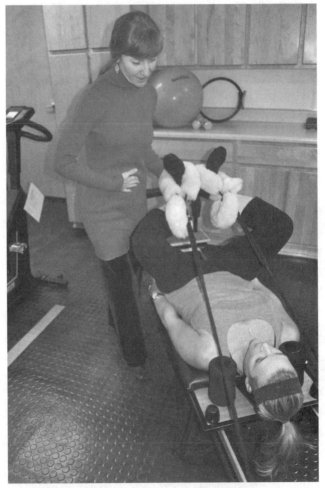

The Frog exercise, *continued.*

Peter Pan Exercise

Although Pilates invented all of the exercises, his successors gave them their nicknames. The Peter Pan exercise, depicted below, is a more advanced exercise. Each leg does something opposing to the other, which requires more coordination and proprioception. Because one leg stretches out to one side, the pelvis wants to tip that way, so Kim must work her core pelvic brace even harder to keep her hips level, to keep from rolling *off* the Reformer, thereby enhancing her balance.

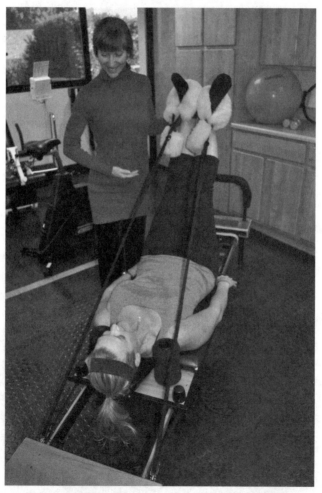

The Peter Pan exercise on a Pilates Reformer.

The Peter Pan exercise is a good example of stretching and strengthening occurring in the same muscle at the same time. Can you see how Kim's right inner thigh is stretching in the photo above? Kim also is strengthening her inner thigh by *holding* her right leg out to the side, as she controls the amount of the stretch (against the force of gravity). The resistance on the cables is kept low and is not enough to fully support her right leg; she must do so by contracting her inner thigh muscles. In the next repetition, she strengthens and stretches the inner thigh muscles of her left leg.

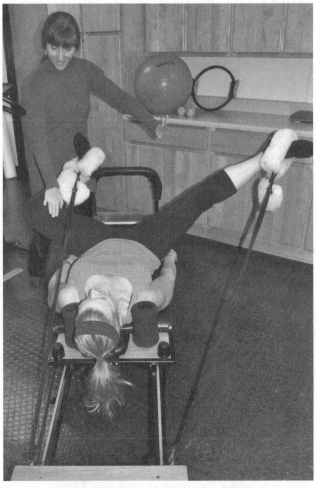

The Peter Pan exercise, *continued.*

Directions for the Peter Pan Exercise on a Reformer:

- Place feet in the large fuzzy stirrups.
- Bring your navel to your spine and squeeze your pelvic floor (the pelvic brace) and hold.
- Start with your legs straight and at 45 degrees (as in the Leg Lower exercise).
- Simultaneously bend your left knee toward your chest as you bring your right leg straight out to the side, knee straight. If you do it correctly, there should be no slack in the cables.
- Return to position in the third step, with both legs straight at 45 degrees.
- Repeat the exercise, reversing your legs.
- Strive to keep your hips level. Your pelvis will want to roll toward the straight leg, but counteract this with your pelvic brace.
- Remember to keep breathing throughout the exercise.

Rabbit Exercise

The formal name for the next Reformer exercise is "Knee Stretch in the Rounded Position." The colloquial name is "Rabbit" (see photo opposite). Can't you just see the resemblance to a little bunny rabbit? This is one example of a kneeling exercise.

Directions for the Rabbit Exercise on a Reformer:

- Kneel on the Reformer and place your hands on the bar. Your toes should be up against the shoulder pads, as shown.
- Curve your spine into a "C" shape, as shown at the right.
- Draw your navel up toward your spine. Squeeze your pelvic floor in (pelvic brace) and *hold*.
- Push the carriage back behind you. Keep your arms still.
- Using your abdominals, draw your legs back under your trunk, returning to the starting position.
- Keep the pelvic brace held tightly.
- Repeat 10 times.
- Remember to keep breathing throughout the exercise.

Plank Exercise

The final Reformer exercise we present is a tough one. Illustrated on page 148, it is called the *Plank* exercise, and it requires great core stamina. Pilates felt that if you could do an exercise correctly three

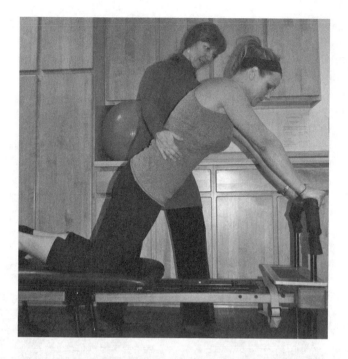

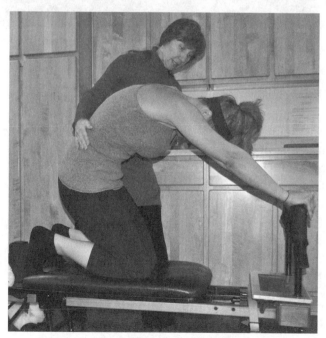

The Rabbit exercise on a Pilates Reformer.

times, it was worth doing, because form and variety are more important than repetitions. Pilates would say three perfect repetitions are better than ten sloppy ones. In the case of the plank, three good repetitions have merit!

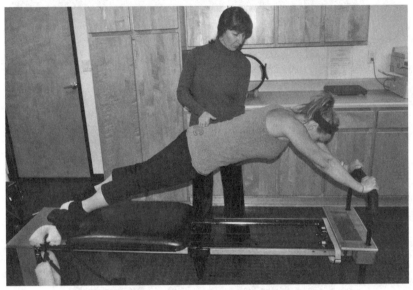

The Plank exercise on a Pilates Reformer.

Directions for the Plank Exercise on a Reformer:

- Start in initial Rabbit position.
- Straighten your legs by pushing the carriage behind you, lifting your knees off the carriage and lowering your pelvis, as shown above.
- Drive your navel up toward your spine and squeeze the pelvic floor (pelvic brace) and *hold*.
- Glide the carriage forward and back, keeping your elbows straight. The only moving joint should be your shoulders.
- Keep your back as straight as a wooden plank. There should be no movement in your back whatsoever.
- Repeat 3 to 10 times, depending on your core stamina.
- Remember to keep breathing throughout the exercise.

You have now gotten a small taste of some common Pilates Reformer exercises. Joseph Pilates created hundreds more! Pilates studios are plentiful in most towns, so consider joining a Reformer

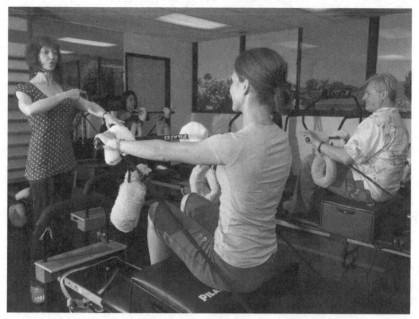

A Pilates Reformer class, showing the Pilates Box and Pole.

class or signing up for private sessions. Ask for a reduced-rate trial session. Many YMCAs also have Reformers.

If you are receiving physical therapy for your incontinence, there is a good chance your clinic has Reformers in its gym, and Pilates can be incorporated into your in-clinic treatment plan. To understand Pilates is to experience it. It's fun!

Pilates Reformer classes are generally quite small (five to eight persons) as compared to larger mat classes (up to 50 persons). In a small Reformer class the instructor will be able to devote more personalized attention to you, giving you easier versions of the exercises and correcting your technique (see photo above).

What if you don't have access to a Reformer? In the next section, we describe some Pilates exercises you can do on almost any flat, slightly padded surface. They mirror three of the Reformer exercises we have just described, only they have been modified into mat exercises.

YOUR HOME PROGRAM WITH MAT PILATES

Pilates mat exercises with small props are beneficial ways to incorporate Pilates into your home program. Not everyone has access or the financial means to enroll in Pilates Reformer classes or take private sessions. In this section we show you some low-cost ways to add a Pilates routine to your life.

The only equipment needed is a yoga-type mat. Ideally, a Pilates mat should be firm and a half-inch thick. A mat that is too thick or squishy will not function well during exercises and will not augment proper balance and alignment. Although a Pilates or yoga mat is recommended, the wonderful thing about mat Pilates is that the exercises can be performed on any padded, level surface, including your carpeted living room floor.

One precaution we must mention here is that your technique must be correct to receive the full benefit and to avoid back or joint injury. There is no substitute for the trained eye of a professional Pilates instructor or a physical therapist. If you take the time to find a class taught by a professional, you can later adapt your knowledge of proper form to your home program and work out on your own. (See Appendix III, page 248, for resources on finding a Pilates instructor.) A video cannot talk back and correct your form.

Mat classes are the most economical way to learn Pilates, because they are offered in group sessions and are usually much larger in size than Reformer classes. Arrive early, and don't be afraid to put your mat at the front of the class. This way, the instructor can see you and give you more cues for correction. You might feel vulnerable as a novice, but doing this will help you learn more quickly and be accurate in your technique. As with Reformer Pilates, mat Pilates has a couple of supporting tools that add "oomph" to a mat routine.

Thera-Bands

Thera-Bands—colorful, rubberized bands—are most commonly used in mat Pilates. These wonderfully inexpensive, portable Pilates accessories consist of wide elastic, and each color represents a different resistance level. Thera-Bands can be incorporated into many different mat exercises to help build muscle strength, tone, and elongation of the muscles.

Magic Circle

Joseph Pilates invented a small piece of equipment called the *Magic Circle* that consists of a thick ring of metal with pads. The original

Magic Circle, circa 1920, was said to have been constructed from the ring of a beer keg by Pilates himself. The mechanics behind the circle echoes Pilates's general theme of adding resistance to help strengthen and define the muscles. The modern day magic circle is about 15 inches in diameter. It consists of a steel ring with a soft rubber covering and padded contoured grips. It can be used to tone all parts of the upper body, including the chest, arms, and shoulders. It can be used for a lower body workout to target the inner and outer thighs, hips, hamstrings, and gluteals. It can be used during both Reformer and mat Pilates exercises and can be added to various Pilates exercises to target and build more core strength. The Magic Circle is easy to work with, portable, and an inexpensive way to boost your Pilates workout.

Below, Kim is squeezing the Magic Circle while holding the table top leg position, with her hips and knees at 90 degrees and her shins parallel to the floor. Many Magic Circles on the market come with educational home videos, making it fairly easy to learn how to use one. (See Appendix IV, page 252, for discount ordering information.)

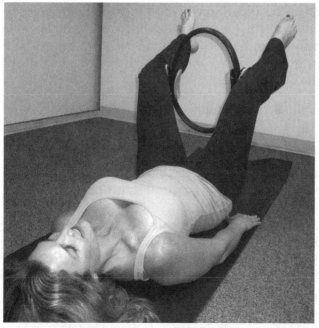

The Magic Circle: Inner Thigh Press exercise.

Directions for the Inner Thigh Press Exercise with the Magic Circle:

- Place the Magic Circle between your thighs, just above the knee joints.
- Draw your navel down toward your spine and squeeze the pelvic floor (pelvic brace) and *hold*.
- Lift your legs into the "table top" position where your hips and knees are at 90 degrees and your shins are parallel to the floor.
- Squeeze the magic circle 10 times.
- Remember to keep breathing throughout the exercise.

Now we will convert three of the Reformer exercises presented in the preceding section into mat exercises you can perform at home: (a) the Hundred exercise, (b) the Frog exercise, and (c) the Leg Lower exercise.

Be aware that even beginner Pilates mat exercises are more difficult than they look. Without the Reformer helping to hold up your legs, your core must work overtime. This is why Joseph Pilates progressed his students to mat exercises only *after* they were proficient on the Reformer. If you pay close attention to the fine details of the following instructions, you should be fine. Do not overdo the repetitions! Good form is more important than a high number of repetitions, so focus on your technique and don't rush through them. Remember to keep breathing throughout your exercise. Keep your pelvic brace engaged during every repetition.

Directions for the Hundred Exercise on a Mat:

- Bring your navel to your spine and squeeze your pelvic floor (the pelvic brace) and *hold*.
- Position your legs as pictured here (this is called the *table top leg position*) with your hips and knees at 90 degrees and your shins are parallel to the floor.
- Stretch your arms long at your sides. Raise your head. (Optional: Lower your head to the mat periodically to rest your core.)
- Pump your hands up and down in small, rapid, six-inch flutters. Keep your elbows straight and your hands relaxed, and strive to make the movement come from your shoulders and shoulder blades.
- Breathe *in* for five little arm flutters and breathe *out* for five little arm flutters.

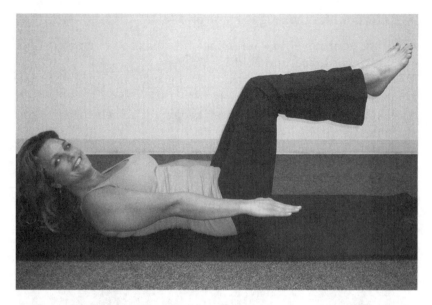

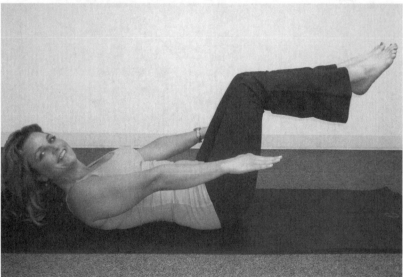

The Hundred exercise, done on a Pilates mat.

- *Do not* allow *any* movement whatsoever in your trunk or back. Don't let it arch. Don't let it flatten. If your lower back arches or flattens, squeeze your pelvic brace harder to disallow movement of your trunk.
- Repeat for 10 breaths and you will have performed 100 little arm flutters. Perform the Hundred once a day.

Directions for the Frog Exercise on a Mat:

- Bring your navel to your spine and squeeze your pelvic floor (the pelvic brace) and hold.
- Assume the table top position. Bring your heels together and toes apart. Squeeze your heels.
- Bend knees toward your chest, keeping the heels together and knees apart, as pictured opposite.
- Straighten your knees out, toward the ceiling, to a 45-degree angle, as pictured below.

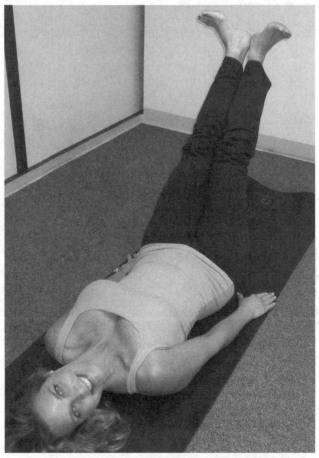

The Frog exercise, done on a Pilates mat.

- Bend your knees again, striving to keep legs moving smoothly on one plane, not wavering up and down.
- *Do not* allow *any* movement whatsoever in your trunk or back. Don't let it arch. Don't let it flatten. If your lower back arches or flattens, shorten the motion and squeeze your pelvic brace harder to disallow movement of your trunk.
- Repeat 10 times, once a day.
- Remember to keep breathing throughout the exercise.
- Optional: Place a loop of a *thin* Thera-Band (red or green) around both feet and hold onto the ends with your hands. This will add some gentle resistance to your legs.

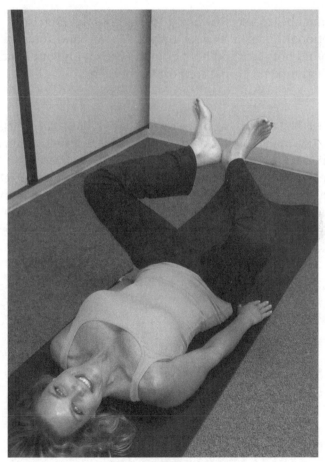

The Frog exercise, *continued.*

Directions for the Leg Lower Exercise on a Mat:

- Bring your navel to your spine and squeeze your pelvic floor (the pelvic brace) and hold.
- Start with your legs high, with your hips at about 90 degrees, as pictured at top left. Squeeze your legs together. Your knees can be slightly bent.
- Slowly lower your legs and *stop* when you feel your back beginning to *arch*, as pictured at the bottom left. This exercise will be much harder without the Reformer supporting your legs, so keep them *high* and move them very little. *Do not go too low!*
- Using your deep abdominals, raise your legs back to your starting position.
- Repeat 3 to 10 times (depending on your core stamina) once a day.
- Remember to keep breathing throughout the exercise.
- Optional: Place a loop of a thick Thera-Band (blue or black) around both feet and hold onto the ends with your hands. This will give some partial support to your legs.

This is just a sampling of the hundreds of Pilates mat exercises that can be done in the comfort of your own home. Self-motivation is often difficult to achieve when exercising on your own, but the gradual reduction of your incontinence and the wonderful postural effects of Pilates will spur you on so you can look and feel better, inside and out.

We, the authors, have personally benefited from years of Pilates training and have seen amazing results in others. Let your hard core overtake your incontinence!

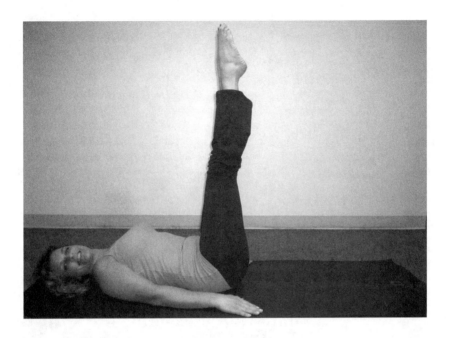

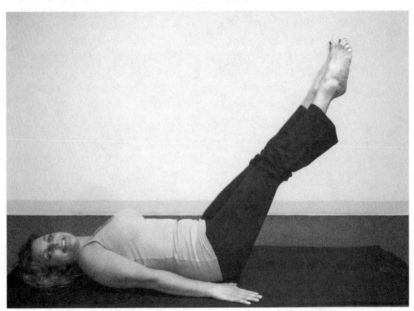

The Leg Lower exercise, done on a Pilates mat.

> "Be faithful in small things because it is in them that your strength lies."
> —Mother Teresa

7 Your Treatment Plan to Support Organ Prolapse

"THE LOWDOWN": MEET ALEXANDRA

I always thought I was so lucky, because my pregnancies were such a breeze. My pregnant girlfriends complained of nausea for months and a diet rich in nothing but soda crackers. I was different. I never experienced morning sickness. Instead, I consumed anything and everything for the entire nine months! I felt full of energy the whole time I was pregnant and never had the sore feet, aching back, or swollen ankles that my friends had. I had three kids, and all three pregnancies went the same way: EASY.

On top of that, I lost my maternity weight in record time, plus an additional twelve pounds within the first year—without even trying! I am someone who has struggled with weight for most of my adult life. Who would have thought having a baby was the answer to my dieting woes? I even dared to feel sexy—trading in baggy sweatpants for tight jeans!

I was getting ready to celebrate my 40th birthday, and I couldn't wait. My husband had planned a very special birthday weekend for me in New York City. We were going to stay in a fancy hotel, see a Broadway show, and spend one special birthday evening with three of my best girlfriends from college and their significant others. I was looking forward to that part of the trip the most, because I hadn't seen those friends in years.

Our plan included a festive birthday dinner followed by dancing at an all-night New York City nightclub. I couldn't wait for my friends to see the new skinny me!

I prepped for the trip for months, and I wanted something really fantastic for the night out with my friends. One day while shopping, I saw a gorgeous pair of black leather pants. Did I dare? Well, I tried them on, and they fit like a glove. I decided to pair them with a sexy (but tasteful) silk blouse, so I didn't look too "Iron Maiden." Instead I felt Vogue *perfect, and I knew my friends would not believe their eyes!*

On another of my shopping excursions, I noticed a weird feeling when I used the department store bathroom. I was sitting on the toilet, doing my typical "speed-peeing" to try to race through my bathroom time (something I habitually did as a mother of three, since there was always someone just outside the door in need of Mommy!) when I noticed a heavy feeling between my legs. It was like something was stuck and needed to get out. I went back into the store and the heavy sensation continued, as if something were pulling from within. I had had that feeling many times before, but that day it was much worse. I felt a nagging, heavy feeling for the rest of that evening.

When I awoke the next day, everything seemed much better. The heavy sensation was there, but to my relief it was much milder. I met my tennis partner for our usual 9:00 match. We had played for about an hour when I suddenly felt the heaviness return full force, and this time it felt like something was literally slipping out of my body. I ran to the bathroom to check and when I felt between my legs there was something hanging out down there. I was motionless. Was I giving birth to an alien? I touched around it and gently tried to push it back inside me. To my surprise, that worked. The whole episode almost made me vomit. I called my doctor from the tennis club parking lot and took the first available appointment.

My doctor diagnosed me with a Stage III bladder prolapse, also called a cystocele. The weight I had felt for so long was the pressure of my bladder sinking lower and lower within my vagina, until finally it slipped outside of my vagina. I wasn't having an alien baby, but that might have been better news. The doctor went on to explain that this was often an after effect of multiple vaginal births. So much for my "perfect pregnancies." She said that I would most likely have this "falling out" experience again and again. She instructed me to be cautious during strenuous activity, which to my chagrin could include walking a lot during the day. I had seen what happened while playing tennis. What was going to happen in a dance club with all of my friends watching?

Later that night, I shared the news with my husband and the options my doctor had discussed with me. Our wonderful trip was just a few weeks away, and I knew one thing for sure: The leather pants were out. I couldn't gamble in my condition, knowing how uncomfortable the tight inseam would feel while dancing, rubbing against my tender bladder if it came out. I might as well pull out my ancient body-camouflaging sweaters and loose pants.

Surgery seemed inevitable. Sure enough, within a year my Stage III cystocele worsened into a Stage IV. The doctor had warned me this could happen, but I did not want to face surgery. Now I had no choice. My prolapse had become so uncomfortable that my doctor suggested I take the first available date for surgery. It had been a year since I was preparing for my birthday celebration in NYC; now I was preparing for surgery. Grudgingly, I scheduled my bladder suspension surgery, which landed within days of my 41st birthday—not exactly the birthday present I had in mind.

Alexandra's story is tragic. The worst part is that she may have been able to do something to stop her prolapse from gaining momentum and moving to life-altering Stage IV. The heavy feeling that Alexandra experienced and became accustomed to should have been addressed long before she got to the point of external prolapse. Her body was trying to tell her something, but she didn't listen. We *must* listen to our bodies and act early to investigate all treatment options. Pelvic organ prolapse is a condition you can't ignore.

Organ prolapse is much more common than you may think. Similar to urinary incontinence, pelvic organ prolapse is an often-closeted condition, but its victims are numerous.

If the embarrassment of your urinary incontinence has not motivated you sufficiently to be conscientious with your pelvic floor exercises, this chapter will. If you are among those who have weak pelvic floors, but no organ prolapse, consider yourself fortunate—and begin doing all you can to create formidable strength in your pelvic floor muscles. If you are already afflicted with organ prolapse, be hopeful: We may be able to help.

TYPES OF ORGAN PROLAPSE DEFINED

PROLAPSE (prō-'lăps)

Slippage of a body part or sinking of a body organ from its usual position, displacement in the body, or a falling out of proper position.

The sensation of organ prolapse is mercilessly uncomfortable. If you are experiencing a feeling of heaviness or pressure in the vaginal area, you may have pelvic organ prolapse to some degree. Organ prolapse occurs when the bladder, uterus, or rectum bulges (or "falls") into the vagina. This creates a most uneasy feeling, similar to what you would feel if a tampon were about to fall out. In the most severe cases, organs protrude completely beyond the vaginal opening, causing many women to panic that they have a cancerous tumor growing "down there." Women often harbor feelings of embarrassment and are reluctant to get medical help until the condition gets considerably worse and harder to reverse.

Like urinary incontinence, pelvic organ prolapse is a very common condition, occurring in thirty-five percent to sixty-five percent of women (American Urogynecologic Society, 2008). It never occurs in men because of the absence of a vagina. Without a vagina, there is no "opening" for organs to fall through. (So much for equality!) The American Urogynecologic Society (2008) reported that approximately 200,000 American women had surgery for pelvic organ prolapse in 2004. In July 2011, the FDA issued a warning against using non-absorbable mesh for bladder sling surgeries due to some adverse side effects (U.S. FDA, 2011). Did you know there is a non-surgical way to improve bladder support?

You have learned in previous chapters that your pelvic floor muscles give you closure strength around your urethra, vagina, and rectum. This is why you have been diligently exercising your pelvic floor muscles—to ward off urinary incontinence. However, the pelvic floor plays another, equally significant role: *support*.

Have you ever seen a model of the human skeleton? Do you remember the large opening at the bottom of the pelvis? Have you ever wondered what keeps your organs from falling out through this large space? It's your pelvic floor muscles. Skin alone would not provide enough support. The bladder, vagina, and rectum rest on the pelvic floor and rely on it for support. When your pelvic floor is thick and well developed, these organs enjoy wonderful support. A strong pelvic floor keeps them in place: high within your pelvis, where they belong. When your pelvic floor muscles are thin and saggy, the organs sag, too.

If your pelvic floor muscles are too weak to hold your organs, the ligaments attached to the organs try to help out. This puts a lot of stress on the ligaments, and eventually they become overstretched and tear. Imagine walking on a rope bridge and, halfway across, the wooden planks underfoot give way. Suddenly, you are left clinging to the ropes. If they fray and start to give, you will fall. Your organs are in the same situation once they lose the support of the pelvic floor muscles. The ligaments can stay intact for only so long without breaking. Finally, they do. Then gravity causes the bladder, the uterus, and/or the rectum to fall into the vaginal space. This can occur intermittently, for example, when the pelvic floor is fatigued after a day of walking at Disneyland, or it can recur daily with any increased intra-abdominal pressure, such as straining with bowel movements.

The diagnosis of organ prolapse is made in two ways. First, the specific diagnosis, pertaining to the organ and the part of the vagina affected, is made. Second, the condition is classified, according to the severity of the prolapse, into stages (I through IV). It is common to have more than one type of prolapse, and it often occurs in conjunction with urinary incontinence. How did we women get this lucky?

In the sections that follow, we identify and briefly describe the various types of organ prolapse women may experience.

Front Wall of the Vagina

This is the most common type of prolapse. When the bladder falls down toward the front wall of the vagina, it is called a *cystocele*. An example of a Stage III cystocele is pictured below. If just the urethral tube, leading from the bladder, pushes into the vaginal space, it is termed a *urethracele*.

Top of the Vagina

Uterine prolapse is when the cervix and uterus (womb) drop down into the vagina. It is the second most common type of prolapse and is the only type in which the organs are actually inside the vagina. In women who have had hysterectomies it is still possible for the vagina itself to collapse, even though the uterus is gone. This is called a *post-hysterectomy vaginal prolapse.*

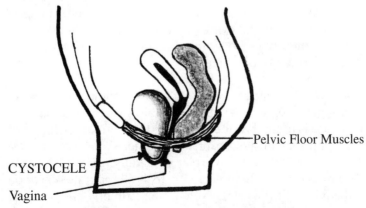

A Stage III cystocele (bladder prolapse).

Back Wall of the Vagina

If the rectum bulges into the vagina, it is called a *rectocele*. This condition may cause discomfort and difficulty having bowel movements. If fecal matter gets trapped inside the rectocele, the woman may have to eliminate it by pushing with a finger from inside the vagina toward the rectum—not much fun, but necessary.

Depending on the severity of the prolapse, the Pelvic Organ Prolapse Quantification system (POP-Q) classifies it as one of four stages. The woman bears down during a *Valsalva Maneuver* (as if to push out a baby or a bowel movement), and a doctor or physical therapist looks into her vagina to check the degree of the prolapse, if any. The same grading system is used for *all* types of prolapse.

Stages of the Pelvic Organ Prolapse Quantification System

Stage 0: This stage represents no prolapse. The bladder, the cervix, and the rectum all stay up where they belong, and no organ movement is observed within the vagina when the *Valsalva Maneuver* is performed.

Stage I: This means that there is virtually no prolapse with the *Valsalva Maneuver*. The bladder, the uterus, and the rectum stay more than 1 cm above the opening to the vagina, as measured from the most severe (lowest) portion of the prolapse. Women have no symptoms with this stage.

Stage II: The bladder, the uterus, and/or the rectum descend but remain essentially within the vagina. This is measured from 1 cm above to 1 cm below the vaginal opening, taken from the most severe (lowest) portion of the prolapse. Women often have no symptoms, or only mild occasional discomfort, with this stage.

Stage III: This stage means that the pelvic organs are beginning to bulge beyond the opening of the vagina. The prolapse is more than 1 cm beyond the vaginal opening but less than the full length of the vagina. When the *Valsalva Maneuver* is finished, the prolapse usually retreats back into the vagina. The patient normally feels a moderate sensation of heaviness in this stage, often intermittently and activity-related.

Stage IV: In this worst case, there is almost complete reversal of the vagina, with the bladder (or other organ) being completely outside of the woman's body. Organs protrude far beyond the vaginal opening, taking the walls of the vagina with it, as if turning a sock inside out. When the *Valsalva Maneuver* is finished, the prolapse often does not retreat back into the vagina, and the organ must be repositioned manually. In this stage, the patient feels a heavy downward-pulling sensation in the vaginal area when standing. It may feel as if she is sitting on a Nerf ball. The prolapse can easily be observed with a handheld mirror.

As you can see, pelvic organ prolapses range from very mild to quite severe. Learning the causes of this condition will be your first step to self-manage your organ prolapse and prevent it from getting worse. We know failed ligamentous support and weakness of the pelvic floor muscles allow pelvic organs to fall and prolapse—but why?

CAUSES OF ORGAN PROLAPSE

There is no single cause of organ prolapse; instead, many factors increase your risk of having mild to severe organ prolapse. These factors relate to the negative impact on the integrity of the pelvic floor muscles, which in turn leads to prolapse.

Childbirth

The major factor causing pelvic organ prolapse is generally thought to be vaginal birth. During vaginal delivery, a woman's pelvic floor muscles have to stretch to the maximum in order for the baby's head and shoulders to pass through the vagina. This may also cause supportive ligaments around the organs to tear. This stretch trauma weakens the pelvic floor considerably. In most women, the damage is minor, but others lose enough muscle integrity that the pelvic floor can no longer hold up the pelvic organs satisfactorily, as was the case with Alexandra.

A 2009 article in the journal *Obstetrical and Gynecological Survey* addressed the relationship between vaginal deliveries and pelvic organ prolapse in 1,350 women (Sze & Hobbs, 2009). Whereas Stage

I or II prolapses did occur more often in women who had had two or more vaginal births, the investigators found that vaginal birth is *not* the major factor predisposing women to Stage III and IV pelvic organ prolapses. The researchers instead concluded that age-related changes produce far more risk of moderate to severe organ prolapse. Maybe this is good news, because who wants to blame severe organ prolapse on one of nature's greatest gifts—the natural birth of our wonderful children?

NOTE: If you are pregnant, or wish to become pregnant, and are experiencing a degree of prolapse, you must remain dedicated to your home program from Chapter 3. This is critical to maintaining your current degree of prolapse or to reversing it a stage. During pregnancy you are more susceptible to further stage progression, so continuing to strengthen your pelvic floor is of paramount importance.

Prolonged Standing/Lifting/Straining

Prolonged standing, lifting, and/or straining can make the bulge larger. Often, the sense of heaviness is worse at the end of the day, when the pelvic floor is fatigued. Conversely, the prolapse may be less apparent on awakening, after the pelvic floor has had a good night's rest in a gravity-free position.

Menopause

Decreased estrogen levels during menopause also may contribute to pelvic organ prolapse. During menopause, collagen and certain connective tissue proteins decline. However, you can regain strength at any age!

Chronic Cough/Smoking

Chronic coughing from smoking, asthma, or chronic bronchitis puts increased and repetitive pressure on the abdomen and pelvic organs. Smoking reduces collagen and can cause tissue deterioration in your pelvic ligaments and muscles.

Incorrect Toileting Body Mechanics/Constipation

Your daily bowel movements can contribute to your chances of developing organ prolapse, or make an existing prolapse worse. Many people hold their breath, push, and strain to evacuate their bowels. This is unwise. Other people, like Alexandra, are in such a rush that they bear down to urinate faster. These practices can lead to organ prolapse, hernias, and hemorrhoids. Not straining, not rushing, and avoiding constipation will help counteract these mechanical factors. Later in this chapter, we teach you correct body mechanics while using the toilet and how to avoid constipation.

Obesity

Obesity increases pressure in the abdomen and makes the pelvic floor work harder in the standing position. Obese women tend to have a forty percent to seventy-five percent higher rate of pelvic organ prolapse (American Urogynecologic Society, 2008); however, not all overweight women are predisposed to this condition.

Hysterectomy

The uterus and cervix have their places in the abdomen, and all of our organs fit like a jigsaw puzzle. It is a widely held belief in the medical community that when the uterus is removed, there is more empty space in the abdomen, increasing the likelihood that the bladder, intestines, or rectum take up this space by falling into it. Because it has lost its innermost attachment, the vagina itself can shorten and collapse downward.

The results of a huge study, Women's Health Initiative Hormone Replacement Therapy Clinical Trial (conducted with a whopping 27,342 women!) did not support this premise, however. The prevalence of cystoceles was 34.3% in women with uteruses and 32.9% in those who had had a hysterectomy. The rate of rectoceles was a virtual tie: 18.6% in women with uteruses and 18.3% in those without uteruses (Writing Group for the Women's Health Initiative Investigators, 2002). So the jury is still out on this issue.

Ethnicity/Race

The Women's Health Initiative Hormone Replacement Therapy Clinical Trial also reported that pelvic organ prolapse is least common in African American women and most common in women of Hispanic descent (Writing Group for the Women's Health Initiative Investigators, 2002). No one is sure why this seems to be the case.

If you have a feeling of increased pressure in your vagina, or you have been formally diagnosed with a cystocele, urethracele, rectocele, uterine prolapse, or vaginal prolapse, this next section was written just for you. Don't resign yourself to discomfort and embarrassment, because there is *plenty* you can do to reduce pelvic organ prolapse!

TREATMENT FOR ORGAN PROLAPSE

If you have a known or suspected case of pelvic organ prolapse, physical therapy can help. It is logical that if weakness of the pelvic floor muscles caused the prolapse, then performing exercises to strengthen the pelvic floor should improve it. Indeed, physical therapy treatment for organ prolapse has been practiced worldwide for decades, with great testimonial success. Robust evidence supporting this intervention has recently become available.

An article published in the *American Journal of Obstetrics and Gynecology* reported that physical therapy for pelvic floor muscle training reversed Stage II or III pelvic organ prolapse by *one full stage* in twenty-two percent of the Norwegian female participants, after just six months of exercise. (The mild cases, women with Stage I prolapse, did not recover to a Stage 0, and Stage IV women were excluded from the study.) Up to 18 in-clinic sessions (with three exercise sessions per day at home) were given to the women. The authors of this study concluded that "Pelvic floor muscle training is without adverse effects and can be used as treatment for prolapse" (Braekken et al., 2010, p. 170).

What gives Braekken et al.'s (2010) study such strong validity is that the prolapse stages were measured with 3-D, real-time ultrasound by clinicians who did not know the group to which any particular woman was assigned (i.e., with or without physical therapy). An even more profound finding is that 74% of the women who received physical therapy noted a decreased frequency of prolapse, and 67% reported less bothersome symptoms. Symptom reduction is the ultimate goal, because significant and troublesome symptoms are the chief indications for traditional surgical intervention. If you suffer with mild to moderate organ prolapse, wouldn't you rather delay—or ultimately prevent—the need for surgery? Noninvasive physical therapy should be tried first.

Rehabilitate Your Pelvic Floor Muscles

Let us now teach you how to build strength, endurance, and co-ordination in your pelvic floor and deep abdominals, in order to reduce your prolapse. Wait a minute! We *already did that*, in Chapter 3! If you follow the physical therapy home program presented there, you will alleviate both your incontinence and prolapse concurrently. If you want to prevent organ prolapse—and who doesn't?—you are already doing so by treating your stress incontinence with the plan outlined in Chapter 3. It's a two-for-one deal!

Incorporate Your Pelvic Brace During Strenuous Activities

You will definitely want to go back and review Chapter 3, because holding the pelvic brace during physical stress is mandatory to im-proving your prolapse and preventing its progression to Stage IV. Because you naturally bear down during activities such as cough-ing, sneezing, lifting, and nose blowing, your organs can slip and make your prolapse worse.

So, you are confidently exercising your pelvic floor in your home program and incorporating your pelvic brace during physically stress-ful daily activities. Good. Now, with some simple daily modifications, you can gain even more protection from prolapse advancement.

Use Correct Body Mechanics
While Moving Your Bowels and Urinating

Yes, you read that heading right. There are correct and incorrect ways to sit on the toilet to pass bowel movements and urine. Even though you have been doing it your whole life, let us impart some toileting education.

Humans have roamed our planet for over 4 million years. Homo sapiens, the species to which we belong, have existed for about 100,000 years. Flush toilets were a luxury when first introduced, and the average family did not have one until the late 19th century. Yet, our anatomy has remained unchanged since ancient times.

For a moment, think of how you would defecate while hiking in the woods without a toilet nearby. You would squat, put your elbows on your knees, and lean forward with your trunk. This is your most natural posture to have a bowel movement (BM). It would prove too difficult and unnatural to sit upright, in a chair-like position, as if you were actually sitting on a toilet seat. You should assume the "hiking in the woods" posture while on the toilet indoors as well! This posture gives a more natural angle to your colon and urethra and adds some safe pressure to the lower abdomen.

Proper Body Mechanics While on the Toilet

■ Sit forward on your toilet. Rest your elbows on your knees, causing your trunk to lean forward. This puts your descending colon and urethra in good anatomical position to empty. These passages have an angle to them (see figure below, which depicts the normal female pelvic anatomy), and leaning forward gives gravity the chance to do more of the work. This posture minimizes the need to strain, which can aggravate your prolapse.

■ By bending forward through the abdomen, you are, in effect, putting safe pressure on your organs. This is far better than a red-faced, breath-holding, prolapse-producing effort to pass that BM!

■ Take your time. Do not rush and add pressure to the process by making your urine or bowel movement come out faster. Let the contractions of your bladder and the peristalsis action of your colon (digestive muscle contractions) do the work.

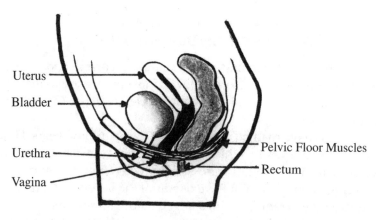

Uterus
Bladder
Urethra
Vagina
Pelvic Floor Muscles
Rectum

The normal female pelvic anatomy.

■ With a difficult BM, breathe out as you apply gentle pressure from abdominal contractions, if necessary. This is the same technique you use when you blow your nose. *Do not* hold your breath and bear down!

Correct Your Constipation

We apologize for causing any squeamishness with such direct talk, but it is important for your continued health that we address bowel function. Whereas it is ideal to have one daily BM, the normal range is from three per day to three per week. Don't think you are abnormal if you skip a day or two. The amount and frequency of one's BMs depend heavily on the types and amounts of food and drink one consumes. Elderly individuals tend to eat less, drink less, and exercise less, resulting in smaller and less frequent BMs.

You want your bowel movements to be soft, thin, and easy to pass. They should resemble a snake and curve in the toilet bowl. If your BMs are shaped more like big hard lumps or pellets, you are probably not getting enough fluid or fiber in your diet. Low fluid intake creates hard, compact stools, because your body wants to keep and use every drop of water you drink, shedding excess fluid only through the BM. Dietary fiber helps the stool retain water, making it softer and easier to pass.

Remember the formula we presented in Chapter 5, to take your body weight and it divide by two? That number—in ounces—is the amount of daily fluid you should consume to meet your bodily needs. It does not have to be all water. Remember, though, that if you perspire through exercise, lose water vapor by talking a lot, or are breastfeeding, you will need to increase your fluid intake accordingly. The following lists contain some suggested nutritional changes you may wish to make, to achieve softer BMs.

Foods That Make Your Stools Softer: ← Eat More

■ High-fiber cereals
■ Whole-meal breads
■ Green vegetables and salad
■ Beans
■ Fruit
■ Nuts

Foods that Make your Stools Firmer: ← Eat Less

- White bread
- Eggs
- Meat

Although many women rely on laxatives, such as Metamucil® and Citracel®, there are more natural, real-food ways to achieve similar results. Make a large quantity of the laxative recipe we offer next. Eat two tablespoons before bed and again in the morning. This will encourage a bulkier, softer bowel movement in the morning. Be patient, because the results will not be apparent the very first night. Stick to this natural dietary supplementation for at least three weeks; it will take time for your system to adjust to the increased fiber. There are no side effects to this yummy concoction!

Recipe for a Homemade, Natural Laxative

1 cup of oat bran
1 cup of applesauce
1 cup of prune juice
- Refrigerate.
- Eat 2 or 3 tablespoons once or twice a day. This can be before bed and in the morning, or at other times of your choosing.

Exercise Regularly and with Low Impact

Do you exercise enough? Some form of daily exercise, done at the same time every day—for example, walking, swimming, or bike riding—will help establish a good BM at a predictable time every day.

You will want to avoid high-impact sports that involve running and jumping, because such activity can aggravate your prolapse (as well as your incontinence). A good guide is that if you need to wear a sports bra during an activity, then it is probably too much for your pelvic organ prolapse as well. Your organs bounce up and down, just like your breasts do!

A super-sized tampon (or two) can add some good vaginal support to your organs if your prolapse is Stage III or less. Tampons fill the vaginal space, so the organs cannot fall into it. This helpful tip came from one of Kathryn's patients who had a Stage III cystocele yet refused to give up her tennis matches. She will be grateful to know her cleverness is being passed on to you!

Pessaries

Unfortunately, Stage IV organ prolapses do not respond well to pelvic floor exercise, because the bladder (or other organs) is already below the level of the pelvic floor. In this fully dropped position, strengthening the pelvic floor will not help much. The only pelvic floor exercises indicated for your Stage IV organ prolapse would be those you perform while lying on your back, after making sure your organs are positioned *above* your pelvic floor. You can even raise your pelvis higher than your head, by putting a cushion from your couch under your pelvis, so gravity can help keep your organs inside. Even with diligent pelvic floor exercise on your back, your organs will probably need more support.

Such support can come from a *pessary*, a small device made of plastic or silicone (similar to a diaphragm) that you or your doctor inserts into your vagina. The purpose of the pessary is to lend extra support to your organs and block them from slipping into your vagina. Pessaries come in many varying shapes and sizes (ranging from two to four inches, see below), and it may take a few trials to

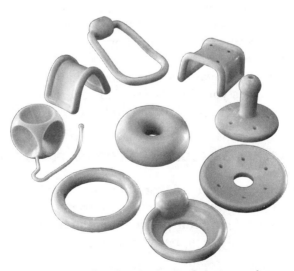

Milex™ pessaries for support of organ prolapse.
Used with permission from CooperSurgical, Inc.

find the one that fits you best and stays in. They are shaped like a ring, a donut, a dish, a cube, or a mushroom.

Either you or your doctor can insert, remove, and clean your pessary weekly, or as infrequently as every few months. Some women have sexual intercourse with the pessary in place, whereas others prefer to remove it. A pessary is an excellent choice if you don't wish to (or cannot) have surgery for a Stage III or IV prolapse. Consult your doctor periodically to make sure the pessary is not irritating your vagina.

Surgical Options

Women with Stage IV organ prolapses that have not responded to pessary support are usually candidates for surgery. A thorough discussion of the various surgical procedures are beyond the scope of this book, and they are highly individualized—for both the woman and the surgeon. Urologists, OB/GYN physicians, and urogynecologists all perform surgical procedures for organ prolapse. Make an appointment with your doctor to fully discuss all of your surgical options.

After surgery, it will be extremely important to fully rehabilitate your pelvic floor muscles, as described in Chapter 3. Bladder suspension surgeries can fail after a period of time, but a strong pelvic floor will help support your organs and increase the chances of a longer lasting postsurgical outcome. Your bladder *still* needs the support from a strong pelvic floor underneath and a strong transversus abdominus muscle in front. Discuss the physical therapy approach with your surgeon before the operation, and ask for a referral for postoperative physical therapy.

For convenience, in the next section we provide an abridged version of the home treatment plan presented in this chapter. Decide which changes you want to make to help reduce and prevent the progression of your pelvic organ prolapse.

YOUR HOME PROGRAM FOR ORGAN PROLAPSE

- **Rehabilitate** Your Pelvic Floor Muscles.
  Follow the comprehensive home program outlined in Chapter 3. The stronger your pelvic floor, the higher it will sit in your pelvis, and the higher your organs will be positioned as well.
- Incorporate Your **Pelvic Brace** During Strenuous Activities.

Remember to contract your pelvic brace during coughing, sneezing, nose blowing, lifting, stair climbing, and any strenuous activity that tends to aggravate your prolapse.

■ Use Correct **Body Mechanics** While Moving Your Bowels and Urinating.
Sit forward on the toilet with your elbows supported on your knees. Take your time. Do not rush the process. Breathe out as you apply gentle pressure, if necessary. *Do not* hold your breath and bear down!

■ Correct Your **Constipation**.
Drink half your body weight in ounces every day. Consume foods high in fiber. Use the recipe given earlier to make a natural concoction of equal parts oat bran, applesauce, and prune juice to use as a natural laxative. Eat two tablespoons, twice a day, adjusting as necessary.

■ **Exercise** Regularly and with Low Impact.
Get daily exercise to avoid constipation and promote bowel regularity. Do low-impact exercise that does not require wearing a sports bra. A super-sized tampon (or two) can add some vaginal support to your organs during exercise.

■ Investigate the Use of **Pessaries**.
If you have a Stage III or IV prolapse, talk to your doctor about a trial with pessaries. Be patient—you will most likely have to try several shapes and sizes to find the one that fits you best.

■ Investigate **Surgical** Options.
If your prolapse is a IV (and pessaries don't work for you), surgery may be your best option. Discuss a postoperative plan of physical therapy with your surgeon, so that your pelvic floor can "relearn" to support your organs effectively. This is critical to ensure the long-term success of your surgery.

Did some of these tips resonate with you? Which lifestyle changes do you believe you should make? We sincerely hope the advice presented in this chapter gives you encouragement and makes a positive impact on the quality of your life.

Discuss your options with your physician. New studies support what physical therapists have known for decades: that physical therapy helps reduce and prevent progression in Stage I, II, and III pelvic organ prolapse. Alexandra was in denial over her symptoms and let them progress all the way to the operating table. Unless you have Stage IV prolapse, it is not too late! Through physical therapy, you may be able to reverse your prolapse an entire stage. Listen to your body, seek physical therapy treatment early, and make surgery your last resort.

> "Adopt the pace of nature: her secret is patience."
> —Ralph Waldo Emerson

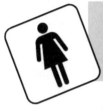

8 Your Treatment Plan for Pelvic Floor Pain and Sexual Issues

"JUST CAN'T DO IT": MEET JESSICA

My wedding was magical, fulfilling my most fantastic childhood dreams. Like most little girls, I began dreaming of my wedding day years before it actually took place. When I was eight, I attended my cousin's wedding, and from that day forward I began planning my own special day.

The ceremony was enchanting. Violins played Pachelbel's "Canon in D" as my father walked me down the aisle of our old family church. I was nervous and excited, realizing that my fantasy was finally real! When I looked down, I noticed the sun was shining through the stained glass windows, creating a kaleidoscope of color spilling over my white gown. It was beautiful. When I looked up, I saw the man whom I loved waiting for me at the end of the aisle, and he was beaming. We were about to begin a wonderful life together.

Believe it or not, this part of the dream came true, far exceeding my girlhood expectations. I had the perfect wedding DAY. My wedding NIGHT, however, proved disastrous.

You see, I was and still am a virgin. I know it's not the "norm" these days to wait to have sex, but for me it was important. Despite my big church wedding, my parents weren't strict about our religion. But from the time I was young, they did teach me the importance of personal values. I can remember my mother's words so well as she advised, "You can lose a lot during your life—your house, your car, your money, but you can't lose your values unless you give them away." This always stuck with me and, as old-fashioned as it was, it was important for me to save myself for my husband. And he was incredibly understanding.

Our wedding day began with such happiness, but it ended in such sadness. I was in tears. They were tears of embarrassment, humiliation, but most of all, pain! I was not naïve enough to believe I was going to experience earth-shattering orgasmic sex during my very first time; however, I did think it would be wonderful to share our love as husband and wife, like we had never done before. Yeah—I was naïve.

The pain was excruciating, beyond anything I had ever felt. The closest experience was when I was thirteen and tried a tampon for the first time. I never did that again. Was sex going to be the same? Pap smears were uncomfortable, too, but I always prepared with some pain medication, and the doctor was very quick. I wish I could say having sex with my husband hurt really badly, yet we still consummated our marriage. I can't say this because we didn't! I couldn't take it!

My husband is the kindest man I have ever met, and you already know he is patient. He was slow, gentle, and caring during our failed attempts. It wasn't his fault, though he kept apologizing. Even partial penetration made me scream, due to the searing pain inside me. We tried everything: different positions, odd angles, and tubes of lubricant. I was willing, just not able.

I have been married now for eighteen months and I am still a virgin. I fear I will never be able to have sex. Besides the relationship with my husband, I want to be a mom. If I can't stand a penis going in—how will I ever live through a baby coming out? What's wrong with me?

Chronic pelvic pain is commonly encountered but rarely understood. According to research published in the journal *Obstetrical Gynecology*, one in seven women has some type of pelvic pain (Mathias et al., 1996), and 39% of reproductive-age women experience pelvic pain with intercourse (Jamieson & Steege, 1996). Ten percent of all referrals to gynecologists are for pelvic pain (Reiter, 1990). Each year, American women spend a horrendous $881.5 million on outpatient visits for this condition, because they usually see multiple specialists before they get an accurate diagnosis (Mathias et al., 1996).

Management of pelvic pain often requires a multidisciplinary approach, and physical therapy is the core of the treatment plan. Andrew Goldstein, MD, director of the Centers for Vulvovaginal Disorders in Washington, DC, and New York City, uses "one simple but powerful word: cure" as he describes "the profound and stunning results" that physical therapists achieve with his patients:

Through the modalities of physical therapy—manipulation, massage, and above all exercises that the patients could do on their own—women who had suffered 'chronic' pain for years stopped suffering. This wasn't just temporary relief from pain. It wasn't palliative. It was a cure. (Stein, 2008, p. ix)

If you suffer from pelvic pain, prepare to receive the cure you have been seeking and to start enjoying life the way Mother Nature intended. Your quest is over.

WHAT IS PELVIC PAIN?

Chronic pelvic pain is defined as nonmenstrual pain inside the pelvis that continues for more than three months. We realize this is a very short, extremely straightforward answer to the question posed in this section title, but the route taken to arrive at the diagnosis of pelvic pain is far from simple. It is a convoluted path, like a mountain switchback, traversed by pelvic pain sufferers who wind through multiple medical pathways trying to find help. All too often, patients feel frustrated because of the frequent dead-ends they encounter in their care. Chronic pelvic pain is a confusing enigma to the medical profession.

In Kathryn's clinical experience, the record for the most doctors a pelvic pain patient had seen was 27. That number is no exaggeration, because the patient's mother kept track! The patient, a vibrant, beautiful, 29-year-old college graduate, had been forced to give up a career she loved, because it required sitting in an office for most of the day. Unable to tolerate the pain of sitting and no longer capable of supporting herself, she moved home to live with her parents. At the time of her first visit with Kathryn, she was in cosmetology school, training to become a hairdresser, because it didn't require any sitting!

This young lady had been evaluated and tested, tested and evaluated (and sometimes treated with medications), by more than two dozen different physicians, but she got no significant relief from her pelvic pain. Twenty-seven different medical doctors (highly respected specialists in their fields) rendered full workups—only to find "nothing wrong." Palliative pain medications gave her some temporary relief but also unpleasant side effects.

Ultimately this woman was referred to Kathryn for physical therapy. The patient's first words were, "If you are going to send me out for another test, I think I will puke right here on the spot. I drove an hour in LA traffic to get here. What are you going to do to actually *help* me?"

This is an example of the high frustration level of pelvic pain patients. Kathryn responded, "The referring stops here. I have nowhere to send you. I won't subject you to any more testing or lab work. Together, let's *fix* this pain." The patient's response was inaudible as tears streamed down her face.

After just twelve physical therapy sessions with Kathryn over three months, the pelvic pain that had lasted ten years was eradicated. The patient could sit again, without slouching back on her tailbone or side sitting on one buttock. She landed a fantastic job in her new field as a hairdresser to Hollywood stars. Gainfully employed, she moved out of her parents' house. She began dating again, because now she could comfortably sit through dinner and a movie. She knew she now had the option of entering a long-term relationship that included intercourse, because it would no longer be painful. She felt whole again for the first time in a decade.

Perhaps we are getting ahead of ourselves. Let's back up for just a minute. The difficult part is that the pelvic floor has a tricky way of referring pain elsewhere—to another body part—often confounding a doctor who is trying to make the diagnosis.

Because of the vast interconnectedness of the human nervous system, the first sign of pelvic floor dysfunction might not be pelvic floor pain at all. The first symptom might be a painful back, thigh, buttock, abdomen, vagina, vulva, bladder, uterus, rectum, or colon, or any combination of those body parts. Thus, patients with pelvic pain may have already seen an orthopedist for the spinal/buttock/thigh pain, an internist for the abdominal pain, a urologist for bladder-related pain, a gynecologist for the vaginal symptoms, a gastrointestinal specialist for the bowel symptoms, and so on. The doctors didn't "miss" the diagnosis, and no one should blame them. Chronic pelvic pain is not well understood and therefore not well managed.

NOTE: Individuals experiencing pelvic pain must see their physicians for full workups, so that life-threatening illnesses (e.g., cancer) can be ruled out.

Most pelvic pain patients are despondent when the doctor says the test results were *negative* (meaning that nothing abnormal was found). Those are dreadful words to any pelvic pain sufferer, because it means no diagnosis and an ongoing, even less hopeful search for pain relief. In frustration, some physicians actually tell patients they must "learn to live with it." Nice medical advice, huh?

How do women describe their pelvic pain? Some of the common adjectives include "burning," "stretching," "tearing," "searing," "sharp as broken glass," "like sitting on a golf ball," or "rubbing against sandpaper." Some women's pain is constant; in others, it varies from day to day, from position to position, and from activity to activity. There might be periods of relative relief, followed by excruciating exacerbations.

The same muscles you have been diligently exercising in the preceding chapters can give rise to extremely painful conditions. This does not mean that exercising your pelvic floor causes pelvic pain; we are just identifying them as the same muscles. In some women, these muscles can get tight, short, and go into spasm, causing extreme discomfort and a loss of function. Any sort of penetration through these pelvic floor muscles (e.g., during sex with your partner, or the insertion of a tampon or a doctor's speculum) can be extremely painful or downright intolerable. Even evacuating the bowels can be a painful, dreaded daily experience.

Let's discuss the causes of pelvic pain so we can get underway with treatment techniques that will make sense!

WHAT ARE THE CAUSES OF PELVIC PAIN?

Which came first, the chicken or the egg? The pelvic floor can be the primary or secondary cause of pelvic pain. Sitting on painful pelvic floor muscles is a common complaint. Did a slouched sitting posture cause tension in the pelvic floor muscles, or did the pelvic floor tension cause the slouch?

There may be some prior conditions that kick-started your pelvic floor pain, yet the pain persisted well beyond the precipitating incident. This can be as common as having delivered a baby vaginally, with the resultant trauma to the pelvic floor and with or without an episiotomy (when the pelvic floor muscles are surgically cut). Pelvic pain could have begun after an annoying urinary tract infection (UTI) but continued long after the infection cleared.

The human body is a complex machine. It is designed to self-preserve, and in doing so it can sometimes compromise itself. Nearby muscles will protect or "guard" around painful body parts, but then pain can develop in these guarding muscles as well. This commonly occurs with shoulder injuries, for example, when the arm is painfully cradled tightly to the chest, causing chronic tension, shortening in the muscles, and soreness in the biceps muscles. Similarly, a painful UTI can make the pelvic floor seize up as the muscles reflexively guard around the pain, causing tension, shortening, and soreness in the pelvic floor, too.

Constantly "holding on" (to prevent accidental urination) due to an untreated case of urinary urgency and frequency can lead to chronic contracting, tightening, and shortening of the pelvic floor muscles. This same overuse and shortening can also occur from stress. Many people have muscle tension in the upper back or neck during times of stress. However, women with pelvic pain carry their tension in their pelvic floors, often clenching these muscles subconsciously.

Here is a brief summary of factors contributing to pelvic floor disorders that can lead to chronic pelvic pain:

- **Trauma:** A fall causing a tailbone (coccyx) fracture; a vaginal delivery; or surgery, such as an episiotomy, hysterectomy, bladder suspension, or C-section can leave the muscles weak and injured. Sexual abuse (especially before age 15) can also lead to chronic pelvic floor pain (Lampe et al., 2000).
- **Muscular conditions:** Weakness and tightness in the muscles of the pelvic brace and trunk may be the problem. Poor posture can wreak havoc in the pelvis. Faulty body mechanics from repetitive lifting or carrying a child on the same hip (the iliac crest of the pelvis) can cause the pelvic bones to shift out of place and tug unnaturally on the pelvic floor.
- **Stress conditions:** The mental stress and chronic clamping of the pelvic floor muscles associated with delaying urination, or the painfully hard stools of constipation, as one tries to "make it to the bathroom in time" can cause a reactive pelvic pain condition. Women who experience pelvic pain often have overwhelming stress in their lives, and they harbor this stress in their pelvic floor muscles.
- **Infection:** UTIs, other bacterial infections, yeast infections, or any major disease in the pelvic organs can precipitate pelvic pain.
- **Inflammation:** Any chronic inflammatory disease in a pelvic organ can initiate a pelvic floor disorder.

A full menu of medical terms is available to diagnose women's pelvic pain conditions, which often carry very similar symptoms.

Female pelvic pain syndromes and diagnoses that can significantly benefit from physical therapy include the following:

- **Pelvic floor tension myalgia:** This is a newer term that consolidates the following syndromes:
  - **Pelvic pain:** Pain in or around the pelvis lasting for three or more months
  - **Levator ani syndrome:** Tightness and tension in the pelvic floor
  - **Coccydynia:** Pain in the tailbone area
  - **Proctalgia fugax:** Severe episodic rectal and sacro-coccygeal (tailbone) pain
  - **Animus:** A malfunction of the external anal sphincter and puborectalis muscle during defecation, including a failure to relax while defecating, causing constipation
- **Dyspareunia:** Painful sexual intercourse
- **Frequency/urgency syndrome:** Severe urge to urinate with constant feeling of fullness in bladder
- **Urethral syndrome:** Swelling of the urethra
- **Vulvodynia:** Pain in the vulva (the external part of the female genitals)
- **Vulvar vestibulitis:** Pain, redness, and inflammation in the vestibule part of the vulva
- **Vaginismus:** Vaginal tightness that causes discomfort and burning pain
- **Interstitial cystitis:** Chronic inflammation of the bladder wall
- **Irritable bowel syndrome:** A disorder that causes abdominal pain and cramping as well as changes in bowel movements
- **Constipation:** Bowel movements fewer than three times a week with stools that are hard, dry, small in size, and difficult to eliminate
- **Diarrhea:** Loose or liquid bowel movements
- **Prostadynia:** A synonym for *chronic pelvic pain syndrome*
- **Pudendal neuralgia:** Irritation and pain of the pudendal nerve (which makes the pelvic floor muscles contract and gives sensation to the external genitalia)

It is extremely difficult to distinguish one pelvic floor pain syndrome from another. Any bowel or bladder disorder may lead to the development of muscle tightening and painful trigger points in the pelvic floor, as well as in the muscles of the lower back, buttocks, and legs. It is no wonder that the medical literature is peppered with articles with titles such as "Chronic Pelvic Pain: Clinical Dilemma or Clinician's Nightmare" (Ghaly & Chien, 2000) and "Pitfalls of the Medical Paradigm in Chronic Pelvic Pain" (Grace, 2000). Doctors are as frustrated as the patients! They receive little to no medical school training on the pelvic floor, and they rarely view it as a treatable source of the patient's pain—until they hear the astonishing results their patients achieve under the care of an experienced pelvic pain physical therapist!

TREATMENT FOR PELVIC PAIN

Physical therapy treatment achieves powerful results in curing musculoskeletal causes of chronic pelvic pain. Andrew Goldstein, MD, boasted that:

> The women [whom I referred to specializing physical therapists] were able to give up their medications that had been controlling their pain, and they were able to return to normal functioning in every way—just by learning to relax and let go of the tension in their muscles, learning to lengthen their muscles, and learning to strengthen their muscles in the right way. (Stein, 2008, p. ix)

Goldstein said he refers 50% of his patients to pelvic floor physical therapists and admits that he "could not be a vulvar specialist without their very important specialty" (Stein, 2008, p. ix). That is strong praise from a physician about physical therapists and the critical role they play in curing pelvic pain!

Like any skeletal muscle, the pelvic floor is capable of getting so tight and so tense that palpable areas of extreme tenderness develop. These trigger points of pain perpetuate and worsen until treatment releases the muscular tension. Physical therapy provides that release.

Have you ever had neck and shoulder tension that seems to start at the base of your skull and radiate to the eyebrow area, giving you a bad headache? Have you noticed the tightness, tension, and soreness in the muscles surrounding your neck, shoulders, and between your shoulder blades? We have all given or received the proverbial neck rub for tension, the kind a boxer gets before he enters the ring. It feels great because the deep massage helps to loosen the tight muscles.

Likewise, each of us has awakened with a stiff neck after a poor night's sleep. With movement and stretching throughout the day, the muscles eventually loosen, and range of motion returns. Stiff and tense pelvic floor muscles are no different; they *crave* and *respond* to massage, stretching, and exercise as well.

Despite the broad smorgasbord of diagnoses floating around, the source of your pain might be traceable to short, tight, tender, hypertonic (i.e., in a spasm) pelvic floor muscles. The natural collaboration of stretching and strengthening exercises, relaxation principles, massage techniques, and breathing exercises we offer in this section will translate into *pain relief*. Ahhhhhhh!

After physical therapy treatment, the elongated, more relaxed pelvic floor muscles can pass bowel movements without pain. The patient can resume sexual intercourse because stretching of the pelvic floor no longer hurts. Women can sit without pain, even on a bicycle seat. Now that the ischemic (blood-starved) areas of the pelvic floor muscles have been nourished through blood-enriching exercise, the pain and tension around the sensitive nerve endings are relieved!

Your home treatment for your pelvic pain comprises the following elements:

- Relaxing and stretching your pelvic floor muscles
- Stretching exercises for the muscles surrounding the pelvis
- External self-massage
- Internal self-massage
- Strengthening exercises
- Behavioral tips
- Relieving stress

The numerous special techniques and exercises presented in this section are taken from the latest medical literature, educational coursework, first-hand experience, and protocols that Kathryn has developed over decades of experience. We have no "cookbook recipe" for you but rather an arsenal of tools that will help you overcome your pain. You must try each one on for size, listening carefully to what your body is telling you. One exercise may feel good, or "hurt good," as is often said in the physical therapy profession. Others may seem to make no difference, and these you can skip. One massage technique will help you successfully locate and release your trigger points, whereas another technique may be too aggressive for your current sensitivity level. Each woman is different, and a good physical therapist tailors her treatment to the patient at hand. You must do the same.

This treatment will take time, because there is no quick fix for chronic pelvic pain. Don't let that frustrate you, because such an attitude will only increase your pain. Instead, be *grateful* there *is* a fix and that you have discovered it. Appreciate every bit of success you achieve along the way to full recovery.

Relaxing and Stretching Your Pelvic Floor Muscles

The typical pelvic floor muscles of patients suffering from chronic pain act differently from the pelvic floors of women with urinary incontinence or pelvic organ prolapse. As you know, with urinary incontinence and pelvic organ prolapse, the pelvic floor is thin, saggy, weak, and in dire need of serious strengthening and toning.

With pelvic pain syndromes, the pelvic floor is restricted, shortened, and tense, and periodically it may even go into spasm. There is too much tone. More than anything else, the pelvic floor needs *relaxation* and *lengthening*. Muscles shorten when they contract, so the pelvic floor does not need more contracting and shortening, at least not in the first phase of rehabilitation.

Why do women with pelvic pain still deal with incontinence if their muscles are so tight? Many people think that a tight muscle is a strong muscle. This is a misconception: A short, tight muscle can still contract, just not very much, because it reaches its state of full contraction (full shortening) very quickly. This does not produce much power at all. For example, if an elbow is already bent at ninety degrees, the biceps can contract only a few degrees farther, producing very little force compared with starting from a straight-arm position. Thus, a short muscle is a weak muscle.

We will teach you some pelvic floor exercises in addition to the ones you learned in Chapter 3 (plus some variations) *after* we have had some success in lengthening and relaxing your pelvic floor. Don't worry if you have already done some pelvic floor exercises. They won't harm you; the blood flow into the muscles is good for them. But at this point, they might not help you.

Surface Electromyographic Biofeedback

How do you relax your pelvic floor muscles? If you were in a physical therapy clinic, the surface electromyographic (SEMG) biofeedback unit would help you learn how to "let go" or "drop" or "release" your pelvic floor muscles. Instead of striving to make the graph go higher when you contract, you would focus on trying to make the graph go *lower* when you are *resting*. This approach is referred to as *downtraining*; in contrast, the strengthening exercises you learned in Chapter 3 are an example of *uptraining*. We will now teach you some at-home ways to relax and lengthen your pelvic floor and thus begin the process of ending your pain.

Learning how to release the tension in these muscles may seem difficult at first. For the muscles to be able to relax, *you* have to relax. It takes some practice, but keep trying and you will succeed. It is imperative for your recovery!

Diaphragmatic Breathing In and Dropping of Your Pelvic Floor Muscles

Breathing, relaxing, and stretching are like three sides of the same triangle acting in harmony. Breathing ensures good oxygenation of your muscles and provides a relaxation response, whereas stretching and dropping both encourage lengthening of your pelvic floor muscles. Let's begin your treatment with learning how to take a diaphragmatic breath.

As you *inhale*, you should see and feel your upper belly rise, as the air flows into your lower lungs because of the action of the diaphragm. Your belly sinks as you *exhale*. Try it a few times.

Doesn't deep diaphragmatic breathing feel relaxing? Deep breathing is a known stress-buster. Sadly, some of us go a full week without taking a single deep, relaxing breath—unless we yawn.

Now add the pelvic floor to your deep diaphragmatic breathing. As you *inhale* and feel the diaphragm move *downward* into your belly, encourage your pelvic floor to follow in the same direction, dropping downward toward your feet. As you *exhale*, the diaphragm and the pelvic floor will both come back up, toward your head.

Allowing your pelvic floor to bulge/drop is similar to the "letting go" you do when you are about to urinate, only not quite to the same degree. The next time you urinate, memorize how this relaxation of the pelvic floor feels, so you can incorporate it into your relaxation training whenever you want.

BREATHE THIS WAY TO ALLEVIATE YOUR PELVIC PAIN

1. **Use your diaphragm:** Place your left hand on your breastbone. Place your right hand on your upper abdomen just below your

ribs. As you *inhale*, you should see and feel your right hand rise up as the air flows into your lungs because of the action of your diaphragm. Your left hand should remain stationary as you avoid putting air into the upper lobes of your lungs. Your right hand sinks back as you exhale.

2. **Relax the tone in your pelvic floor**: Imagine that your abdomen, waist, and pelvic floor are expanding like a beach ball being inflated. As you draw the air *in*, your belly and waist bulge *out* as your pelvic floor simultaneously bulges *down*, as the "ball" gets larger in all directions. Try it again, breathing *in* for five seconds, then breathing and bulging *out* for five seconds.

Hold a mirror up so you can watch yourself relax your pelvic floor. The rectum should bulge and open, as if you were to pass gas or a bowel movement. The space between your rectum and vagina (the *perineal body*) should also move toward the mirror as your muscles descend with inhalation.

Another good cue is to try and imagine your sit bones (*ischial tuberosities*) moving away from each other, as the space between them broadens with your slow deep breath in.

You may have to reread and repeat these instructions over and over until you "get it," because this relaxation technique is *very subtle*. Don't expect huge movement. The tension has existed in your pelvic floor muscles for a very long time, and it will take diligence to learn how to eliminate it. You may not have even realized that those muscles were tense before you read this book!

Now let's add some stretching exercises for the pelvic floor, coupled with the deep breathing and dropping/bulging technique. This will relax your pelvic floor more effectively. Try all three stretch positions to see which one works best for you, based on your pain level and flexibility. On the next three pages, coauthor Kathryn Kassai, PT, demonstrates the exercises.

Try stretching and relaxing your pelvic floor muscles on a chair (or a large physio-ball if you have one), as shown on page 200. Take a few diaphragmatic breaths, then, on the next breath in, drop and bulge your pelvic floor down onto the chair. Did you feel the pelvic floor muscles drop downward as you breathed in? Good! You are learning to lose the tension in your pelvic floor muscles! Keep practicing this intermittently throughout the day, every day. It is best to *not* let the stress of daily life build up and take residence in your pelvic floor. If you find yourself in a stressful situation at work or at home, do one of these next three exercises at your first opportunity.

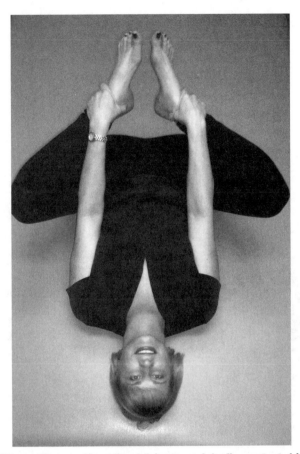

"Squatting on Your Back" (easy pelvic floor stretch).

INSTRUCTIONS: This is the easiest way to begin stretching your pelvic floor muscles. Assume this stretch position. Take two relaxing diaphragmatic breaths, and notice how your belly expands as you take the air into your lungs. Inhale and exhale for five seconds each. On the third breath in, allow and encourage your pelvic floor to bulge or drop downward (toward your toes) as the air fills your trunk. Keep breathing in and bulging downward, while you hold this stretch for 60 seconds (or two stretches of 30 seconds).

CAUTION: Do not do a *Valsalva Maneuver* by holding your breath, then bearing down to *make* your pelvic floor muscle bulge downward as you exhale. We purposely are asking you to bulge or drop the pelvic floor as you inhale, so the *Valsalva* cannot play a part in these exercises.

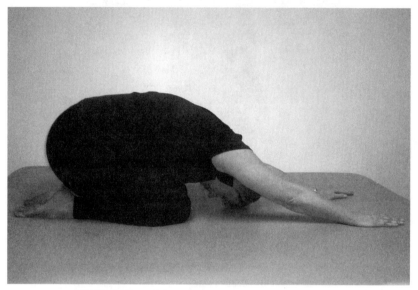

"Child's Pose" (moderate pelvic floor stretch).

INSTRUCTIONS: This exercise provides a moderate stretch of your pelvic floor muscles. Assume this stretch position. Take two relaxing diaphragmatic breaths, and notice how your belly expands as you take the air into your lungs. Inhale and exhale for five seconds each. On the third breath in, allow and encourage your pelvic floor to bulge or drop downward (toward your toes) as the air fills your trunk. Keep breathing in and bulging downward, while you hold this stretch for 60 seconds (or two stretches of 30 seconds).

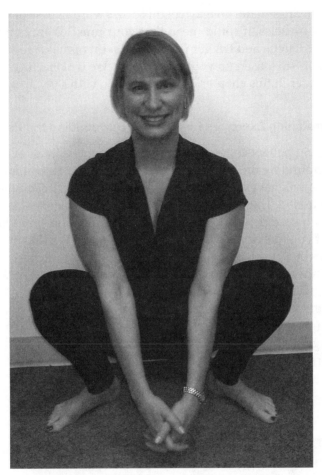

"Frog Squat" (difficult pelvic floor stretch).

This is the most challenging—but most effective—way to stretch your pelvic floor muscles. Assume this stretch position. Put your forearms on your thighs and gently press your elbows outward. Take two relaxing diaphragmatic breaths, and notice how your belly expands as you take the air into your lungs. Inhale and exhale for five seconds each. On the third breath in, allow and encourage your pelvic floor to bulge or drop downward (toward your toes) as the air fills your trunk. Keep breathing in and bulging downward while you hold this stretch for 60 seconds (or two stretches of 30 seconds). **OPTIONS:** Lean against a wall for added balance and support, or place a small footstool underneath your buttocks to support yourself in a partial (instead of a full) squat position.

CAUTION: Omit this exercise if you have knee problems or pelvic organ prolapse, or if you lack the flexibility in your legs.

If you are still not able to feel this downward release of your pelvic floor muscles, it could mean that your muscles are bound tight with restrictions and trigger points, and a bit of massage should be done first—to loosen up your pelvic floor. We will teach you how to do this later in this chapter. Hang tight—or, better yet, hang loose!

Stretching Exercises for Muscles Surrounding the Pelvis

Pelvic pain patients often have muscular tightness in all of the muscles surrounding the pelvic floor. Stretching other skeletal muscles in this zone will have an overflow tension-relieving effect on the pelvic floor muscles. These neighboring muscles may be sites of referred pain from your pelvic floor, or the muscles might be "guarding" because of your pelvic floor pain. They need stretching in either case. All stretches in this section will be held for 60 seconds (or two stretches of 30 seconds) and will be combined with a deep breath *in* at the same time you *bulge* or *drop* your pelvic floor muscles.

Kathryn demonstrates six exercises, pictured here, but we are not suggesting that you do them all routinely. Select three or four that target the areas where you feel the most tightness, and perform them once a day.

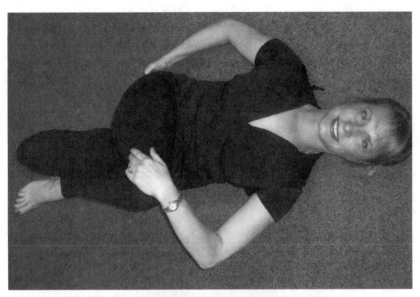

"Pretzel Stretch."

INSTRUCTIONS: This stretch is for a deep buttock muscle that rotates your hip joint in an outward direction (called the *piriformis muscle*). Assume this stretch position. Do not twist your back. Take two relaxing diaphragmatic breaths, and notice how your belly expands as you take the air into your lungs. Inhale and exhale for five seconds each. On the third breath in, allow and encourage your pelvic floor to bulge or drop downward (toward your toes) as the air fills your trunk. Keep breathing in and bulging downward while you hold this stretch for 60 seconds (or two stretches of 30 seconds). Repeat with your left leg crossed on top. **OPTION:** Massage and release your piriformis muscle by pressing your knuckles deep into your buttocks where you feel the stretch and the tenderness.

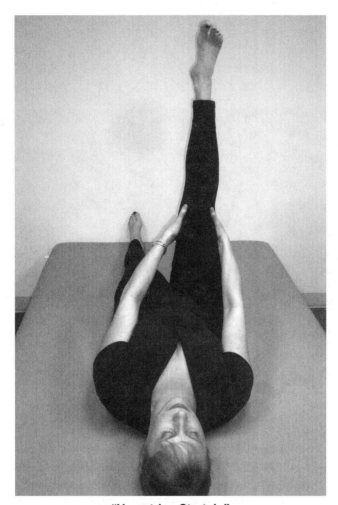

"Hamstring Stretch."

INSTRUCTIONS: Assume this position to stretch the backs of your thighs. Keep your knee as straight as possible. Take two relaxing diaphragmatic breaths, and notice how your belly expands as you take the air into your lungs. Inhale and exhale for five seconds each. On the third breath in, allow and encourage your pelvic floor to bulge or drop downward (toward your toes) as the air fills your trunk. Keep breathing in and bulging downward while you hold this stretch for 60 seconds (or two stretches of 30 seconds). Repeat with your left leg toward the ceiling.

OPTION: If you can't comfortably reach your knee, you can use a rope or a bathrobe belt. Place the rope or belt around the arch of your foot and hold the ends with your hands. This will support your leg as you stretch your hamstrings. Remember to keep your knee straight.

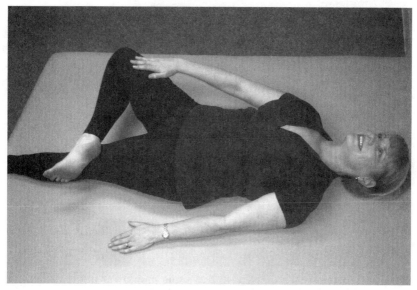

"Figure 4 Stretch" (inner thigh).

INSTRUCTIONS: This stretch is for the inner thigh (the hip adductor muscles). Assume this stretch position. Take two relaxing diaphragmatic breaths, and notice how your belly expands as you take the air into your lungs. Inhale and exhale for five seconds each. On the third breath in, allow and encourage your pelvic floor to bulge or drop downward (toward your toes) as the air fills your trunk. Keep breathing in and bulging downward while you hold this stretch for 60 seconds (or two stretches of 30 seconds). Repeat with your left leg bent and open to the side.

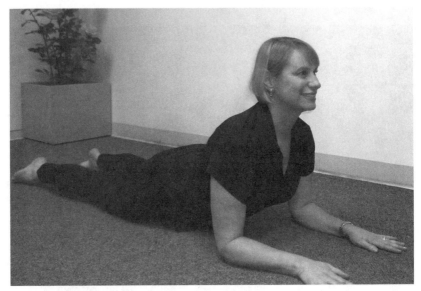

"Sphinx Stretch" (for abdominals and lower back).

INSTRUCTIONS: This exercise simultaneously stretches the abdominal muscles and the lower back. Assume this stretch position. Lift your head and trunk to the ceiling until a comfortable stretch is felt in the back. Take two relaxing diaphragmatic breaths, and notice how your belly expands as you take the air into your lungs. Inhale and exhale for five seconds each. On the third breath in, allow and encourage your pelvic floor to bulge or drop downward (toward your toes) as the air fills your trunk. Keep breathing in and bulging downward while you hold this stretch for 60 seconds (or two stretches of 30 seconds).

CAUTION: Omit this exercise if it aggravates your back.

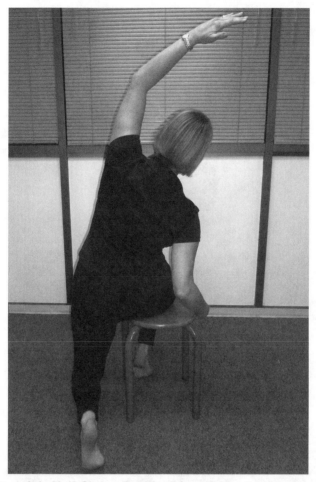

"Side Stretch in Half-Sitting Position" (*quadratus lumborum* **muscle).**

INSTRUCTIONS: You will need a chair without armrests for this exercise. As pictured, this stretching exercise targets the left side of your trunk and waist. Assume this stretch position. Notice that Kathryn is sitting with only her right buttock on the chair, allowing her left buttock to drop down. Side bend to the right until a comfortable stretch is felt on the left side of your waist. Hold onto the chair for support. Take two relaxing diaphragmatic breaths, and notice how your belly expands as you take the air into your lungs. Inhale and exhale for five seconds each. On the third breath in, allow and encourage your pelvic floor to bulge or drop downward (toward your toes) as the air fills your trunk. Keep breathing in and bulging downward while you hold this stretch for 60 seconds (or two stretches of 30 seconds). Repeat on the other side.

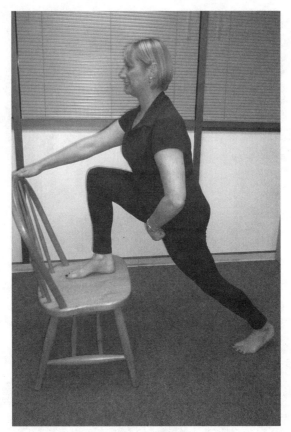

"Hip Flexor Stretch" (*iliopsoas* **muscle**).

INSTRUCTIONS: You will need a chair with a back for this exercise. This stretch is very important for anyone who sits a lot, because extended periods of sitting can cause the muscles in the front of the pelvis and hip joint (the iliopsoas muscle, or *hip flexors*) to become short and tight. Assume this stretch position. It's OK for your left knee to bend a little, and be sure you tuck your tailbone under to flatten your back—you will feel a stronger stretch this way. Take two relaxing diaphragmatic breaths, and notice how your belly expands as you take the air into your lungs. Inhale and exhale for five seconds each. On the third breath in, allow and encourage your pelvic floor to bulge or drop downward (toward your toes) as the air fills your trunk. Keep breathing in and bulging downward while you hold this stretch for 60 seconds (or two stretches of 30 seconds). You can rotate your pelvis in little circles to feel different fibers stretching. Reverse leg and arm positions and repeat.

OPTION: Use your knuckles to massage and release the muscles you are stretching (at the front of the hip joint).

External Self-Massage

A pelvic floor physical therapist will massage your pelvic floor externally in order to ease the muscle tension. Several examples of external self-massage are depicted on pages 200 through 206.

Trigger points are tender knots in the muscle that can refer pain elsewhere. It will "hurt good" to deactivate trigger points, just as it would if they were located in the upper trapezius muscles between your neck and shoulders. The physical therapist also will want you to use similar techniques at home to promote faster recovery. By applying various types of self-massage and trigger point release techniques, you can further lengthen and relax your pelvic floor muscles at home. All of these external self-massage techniques can be performed fully clothed, as long as the garment is loose and thin enough to enable you to feel the massage.

In the first technique, a large physio-ball (also called a *Swiss ball* or a *gym ball*) is used. These balls come in four sizes and can be purchased at any sporting goods store.

HOW TO BUY THE CORRECT SIZE PHYSIO-BALL

When you stand alongside a physio-ball, the top of the ball should be slightly above your knees. When you sit on a fully inflated ball, your knees should be bent at 90 degrees, and your thighs should be parallel to the floor. Here is an approximate sizing chart, based on your height:

Height:	Ball Size
Under 5 ft	45 cm
5 ft → 5 ft, 5 in.	55 cm
5 ft, 6 in. → 5 ft, 11 in.	65 cm
Over 6 ft	75 cm

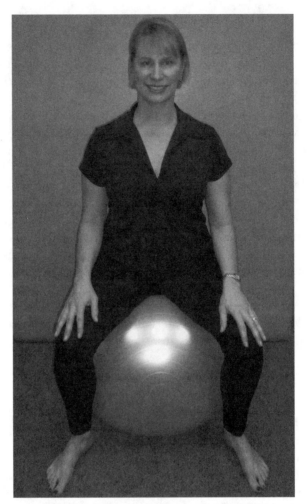

"Bounce and Gyrate" on a physio-ball.

INSTRUCTIONS: You will need the proper-sized (i.e., for your height) physio-ball for this exercise. The curvature of the ball will press up and into your pelvic floor, thereby stretching it. Your pelvic floor will welcome the overall stretch provided by the ball's contact pressure. First try bouncing up and down while on the ball. You should feel a rhythmic release of your pelvic floor muscles. Next try shifting your pelvis right, left, forward, and back on the ball. Now make gyrating circles with your pelvis clockwise and counterclockwise, as you appreciate the gentle massaging effect this exercise brings. Keep breathing and continue bouncing and shifting for several minutes. It's fun!

OPTION: If your balance is poor, wedge the ball in the corner of your room. This will keep the ball stationary. Releasing some air from the ball will also make it more stable.

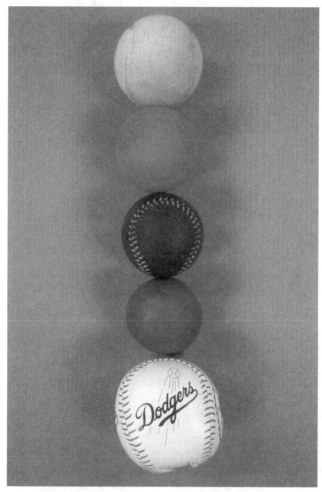

Collection of small balls for progressive self-massage of the pelvic floor

INSTRUCTIONS: You may want to buy an inexpensive collection of small balls, because they make useful tools to self-massage your pelvic floor. Here they are displayed in order from softest (bottom) to hardest (top). The "Dodger" ball is super soft and collapses nearly flat with pressure. (GO Dodgers!) The second ball from the bottom is a "stress ball" filled with contouring seeds—most sporting goods stores carry these balls. The next ball is a soft, indoor foam baseball that toy stores carry. Second from the top is an old-fashioned, dime-store, pink, bouncing ball, and the most firm is the common tennis ball at the top of the photograph.

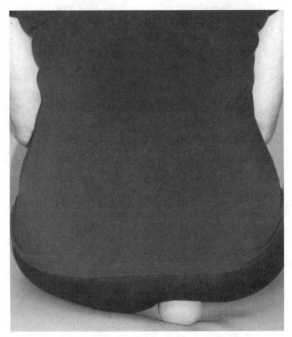

"Small Ball Massage" of the pelvic floor.

INSTRUCTIONS: Start with the softest ball in your collection. Place it just inside of your right sit-bone (*ischial tuberosity*) and sit on it. Let the convex curvature of the ball press up and into your pelvic floor, thereby stretching it. Try shifting right, left, forward, and backward on the ball in order to find your tender trigger points. Once you find a tender point, hold the pressure for 30 to 90 seconds until the tenderness lessens or disappears. Add your deep diaphragmatic breath in as you let go and allow your pelvic floor to melt down around the ball for further stretching and relaxation. Reposition the ball on the inside of your other sit-bone and compare sides. Next, place the ball in the center of your pelvic floor, on the space between your rectum and your vagina (called the *perineal body*). Continue finding new trigger points as tolerance allows. Keep breathing and relaxing your pelvic floor.

PROGRESS: Increase your self-massage by graduating to firmer balls that give you some discomfort but not pain. Realize that the firmer the chair, the more pressure you will feel. A soft couch will absorb the ball, lessening the pressure, and this is OK, because your pelvic floor may not tolerate much pressure initially.

OPTION: For a more aggressive stretch, do a 10-second pelvic floor contraction while sitting on a small ball. The area of your pelvic floor that is being stretched over the ball will try to shorten with the contraction, but the ball will block this shortening, stretching the pelvic floor muscles where you need it most. Afterward, do a deep breath in as you drop your pelvic floor over the ball for a final relaxation.

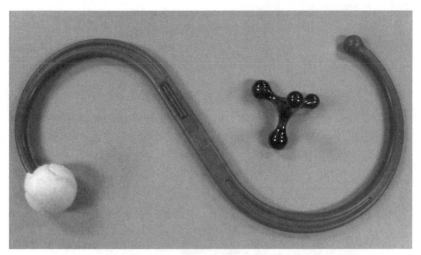
Backnobber® and Jacknobber® self-massage tools.

INSTRUCTIONS: You may want to invest in these two items, because they are indispensable for self-massage and work the trigger points in your pelvic floor and elsewhere. Some areas of the body are difficult to reach, and the Backnobber® solves this problem. These tools provide more aggressive self-massage and trigger point release because they are made of hard plastic. The Backnobber® comes apart at the middle, making it easy to take both tools when you travel. Discount ordering information is provided in Appendix IV, page 252.

OPTION: Soften and distribute the pressure by putting a scored tennis ball on one of the knobs.

HOW TO APPLY PRESSURE TO A TRIGGER POINT

Practice this on a tender point in your forearm muscles to get the idea. Apply gentle pressure with your thumb, finger-tips, or a massage tool, and slowly add pressure until you rate the discomfort as a "5" on a 1-to-10 scale (with 10 representing the most severe discomfort). Hold this pressure and *wait* patiently for thirty to ninety seconds for the soreness to reduce down to a 2 or 3. Then add a little more pressure, bringing the discomfort back to a level 5, and hold for another 30 to 90 seconds until the tenderness reduces again. You are "pushing" the soreness away but never causing yourself actual pain that could cause the muscle to react and go into spasm. Lift your finger off the trigger point slowly. You will be amazed how well this works!

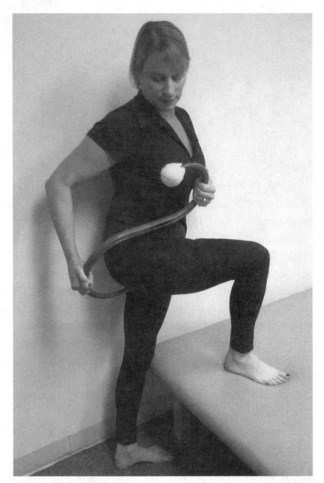

Use of the Backnobber® to massage the pelvic floor.

INSTRUCTIONS: Assume the above position. Place the Backnobber® inside one of your sit bones and gently lift up to apply tolerable pressure around it. Hold the pressure for 30 to 90 seconds until the soreness melts away. Reposition the Backnobber® on the inside of your other sit-bone and compare sides. Next, place the Backnobber® in the center of your pelvic floor, on the space between your rectum and your vagina. Continue finding new trigger points as your tolerance allows. Keep breathing and relaxing your pelvic floor as you massage.

OPTION: Use your Backnobber® on your mid and lower back, gluteals, waist, upper back between your shoulder blades (a favorite spot), on your upper trapezius muscles, and any other place needing a massage!

CAUTION: Don't overdo it, or you will be sore the next day. "Less is more" with the Backnobber®.

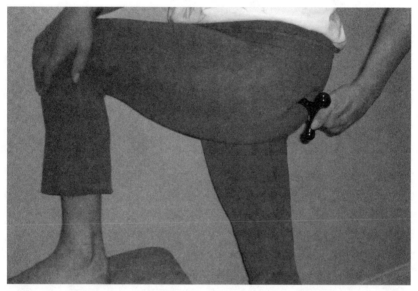

Using the Jacknobber® to massage the piriformis and buttock muscles.

INSTRUCTIONS: The Jacknobber® is a smaller, more affordable version of the Backnobber® and is useful if the muscle is easy to reach. Use it on your buttocks (as pictured) and inner thighs to find common trigger points associated with pelvic floor pain.

OPTIONS: With your other hand, draw your thigh inward to give a better stretch (as pictured), or use your Jacknobber® on your inner thighs, hip flexors, and any other place that needs a massage!

CAUTION: Don't overdo it, or you will be sore the next day. "Less is more" with the Jacknobber®, too.

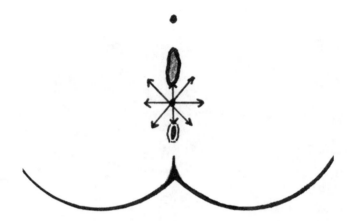

External "Snowflake" massage (of the perineal body).

INSTRUCTIONS: Refer to page 36 in Chapter 2 to locate the space between your rectum and your vagina. Do you see how most of the pelvic floor muscles seem to converge there? This is called the *perineal body*, but it is really just a reference point within the pelvic floor muscle. Without a doubt, this is the *most tender* spot in the pelvic floor. Episiotomies cut into this area of the muscle, and intercourse stretches this region. Use a hand mirror to help you find your perineal body. Then put on some stretchy leggings or thin sweatpants. Lie on your back with knees bent and apart. Place your middle finger on your perineal body. Apply and hold some pressure for 30 to 90 seconds, until the soreness melts away. Maintain this pressure and draw your finger upward, gliding the perineal body for a massaging stretch. Hold for 30 seconds (or as tolerable) and repeat in all directions as shown above, making a "snowflake" pattern. You control the amount of massage pressure and stretch. Be sure to keep it tolerable and in the "hurts good" descriptive category.

OPTION: You can also make little circling motions on your perineal body with your finger.

Internal Self-Massage

Up to this point in the chapter, we have presented a medley of ways to stretch, relax, and massage the pelvic floor muscles externally. Now it is time to work inside. You may feel apprehensive reading this next section, because it involves mobilizing inside your vagina to stretch and massage your pelvic floor muscles. Please do not shy away, however, because this is a necessary element for your recovery. The massage you give yourself will lengthen the soft tissues of your pelvic floor, deactivate the tender trigger points in your muscles, and increase the blood flow, as tension-causing toxins are carried away—taking your pain with it!

You will be placing your thumb inside your vagina. You can wear latex-free examination gloves if this makes you more comfortable. Instead of your thumb, you can obtain the smallest medical dilator, as pictured on page 210. You will give yourself this massage in the privacy of your own home at a relaxing time in your day.

Although the massage techniques you will learn in this section will be gentle, the initial contact can create a burning sensation. This is a normal, desired effect that will subside after a short time. In fact, this is a sign that you *need* these massaging and stretching techniques. Realize that none of these techniques are painful for women who don't have pelvic pain. Soon you will be one of them!

Try to relax your mind completely while you do these exercises. Get comfortable. You may want to darken the room or play your favorite slow song on your iPod. You can even do these self-massaging stretches in the warm water of your bathtub, surrounded by candles. Look at it this way: If you are (or wish to be) sexually active, these techniques are mandatory to returning to pain-free intercourse. If you aren't sexually active, then becoming pain-free is your motivational force. These positive goals should drive your motivation and help overcome any reluctance you may have.

According to Amy Stein, physical therapist and author of the book *Heal Pelvic Pain: A Proven Stretching, Strengthening, and Nutrition Program for Relieving Pain, Incontinence, IBS, and Other Symptoms Without Surgery*, "Where your pelvic floor disorder is concerned, massage is (also) an essential tool of the healing process" (2008, p. 88). Of course, your other option is to ask your doctor for a referral to a physical therapist who specializes in Women's Health and treats pelvic pain. She can perform soft tissue mobilization and teach you how to do it. She also can give you a comprehensive tailored program that is directly applicable to your pain.

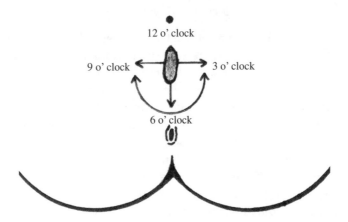

"Clock" and "Smile" internal thumb massages.

INSTRUCTIONS: Put on latex-free exam gloves if you wish. Get into a semisitting position in bed, with pillows supporting your back. Bend your knees and open them. Apply some water-soluble lubricant (K-Y Jelly® or Slippery Stuff®) to your thumb. Do a pelvic floor contraction and feel your perineum lift toward your head and then relax back to its resting position. Squeeze again, and this time, slowly insert your thumb *while* you are relaxing. This is the least painful moment to insert your thumb. If it takes three pelvic floor squeezes and relaxations before you get your thumb two-thirds of the way into your vagina, that is fine. Here is the progression of techniques now that you are "in":

(a) Breathe and relax. As you learned throughout in this chapter, take a deep breath in as you allow your pelvic floor to bulge or drop down. Take three breaths and relax your pelvic floor more with each one. Feel the relaxation of the pelvic floor and the desensitization of your nerve endings, as your vagina gets used to having your thumb inside.

(b) Visualizing the "clock" shown here, gently press your thumb downward, toward the 6 o'clock position (toward your perineal body). Hold for 60 seconds as you stretch your pelvic floor muscles. You may feel a burning sensation as the tissues stretch. This is a desired, normal effect and it should subside after a short time. Move your thumb toward 3 o'clock, stretch, and hold for 60 seconds again. Repeat the same at the 9 o'clock position, taking note of which side is more tender. Usually one side of the vagina is more painful than the other. You will *not* press toward 12 o'clock because this will feel uncomfortable on your urethra.

(continued)

(c) Make a "smile" motion as you press and sweep your thumb between 9 o'clock and 3 o'clock. Add as much pressure as you comfortably tolerate. Pause and hold the stretch at any point along your "smile" that you feel is especially tender. Keep breathing and relaxing your pelvic floor muscle. Do not tense up and work against yourself. Try doing six slow "smile" sweeps, and put a smile on your face as well!

OPTION: For a more advanced stretch, repeat step (b), but add a gentle 10-second pelvic floor squeeze around your thumb. Try to maintain the outward pressure of your thumb (into the 3 o'clock, 6 o'clock, and 9 o'clock positions) as you squeeze. After you relax, see if you can press your thumb into your pelvic floor a little further, taking up the slack in the muscle you just created. Repeat the squeeze three times at each clock position, or at any place along your "smile" where you feel soreness and tightness.

We know that the items pictured on page 210 look like they came from a sex shop. They are vaginal dilators, manufactured and distributed by a highly respected medical company, Syracuse Medical. Physical therapists are eternally grateful for these dilators, because they are invaluable for stretching the pelvic floor muscles around the vagina, training for pain-free sexual intercourse, or providing general pelvic pain relief. Physical therapists couldn't do their jobs without them.

A set of vaginal dilators contains four (to seven) progressive sizes; your physical therapist will order the correct size for you. They are very smooth and made of medical-grade, non-latex, rigid plastic. The smallest vaginal dilator can be used to replace your thumb for the "clock and smile" massage technique that begins on the previous page. The medium to large dilators will progressively and gently enlarge your vagina and pelvic floor until you are pain free with the largest one. Once you can tolerate the large dilator, you'll know you are ready to receive your partner's penis and return to pain-free (and eventually enjoyable) sex. Jessica will be overjoyed when she reaches this stage in her home program!

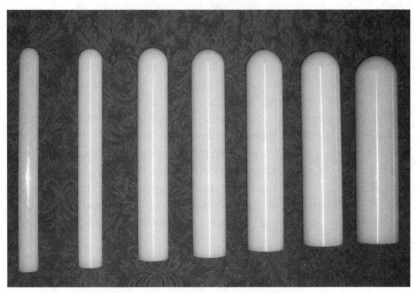

Stretching with vaginal dilators.
Used with permission of Syracuse Medical.

INSTRUCTIONS: Lie on your back with your knees bent and apart with your head partially elevated. Apply some water-soluble lubricant (K-Y or Slippery Stuff) to the smallest dilator. Do a pelvic floor contraction and feel your perineum lift toward your head and then relax back to its resting position. Squeeze again, and this time, slowly insert the dilator *while* you are relaxing. About three inches should remain outside, and you will grasp this section with your hand. Relaxing after a pelvic floor contraction will be the least painful moment to insert your dilator. Don't worry if it takes three pelvic floor squeezes and relaxations before you get your dilator inserted. Take your time and do not rush. Here is the progression of techniques now that your dilator is "in":

(a) Breathe and relax. As you have learned throughout this chapter, take a deep breath in as you allow your pelvic floor to bulge or drop down. Take three breaths and relax your pelvic floor more with each one. Feel the relaxation of the pelvic floor and the desensitization of your nerve endings as your vagina gets used to having the dilator inside.

(b) With the dilator in the center of your vagina, squeeze your pelvic floor muscles for 10 seconds around the dilator. The muscle fibers are trying to come together, but the dilator is blocking them, so some wonderful stretching results.

(c) Alternate each squeeze with your breath in and drop/bulge technique as described in step (a). Repeat five cycles.

(*continued*)

(d) Visualizing the "clock" from page 208 and gently press the dilator downward, toward the 6 o'clock position (toward your perineal body). Hold for 60 seconds or as tolerated as you stretch your pelvic floor muscles. Move the dilator toward 3 o'clock, stretch, and hold for 60 seconds again. Repeat the same with 9 o'clock, taking note of which side is more tender. Usually one side of the vagina is more painful than the other. You will *not* press toward 12 o'clock because this will feel uncomfortable on your urethra.

(e) Make a "smile" motion as you sweep your dilator between 9 o'clock and 3 o'clock. Add as much pressure as you tolerate comfortably. Pause and hold the stretch at any point along your "smile" that you feel is especially tender. Keep breathing and relaxing your pelvic floor muscle. Do not tense up and work against yourself. Try doing six slow "smile" sweeps.

OPTION: For a more advanced stretch, repeat step (b), but add a gentle 10-second pelvic floor squeeze around the dilator. Try to maintain the outward pressure of the dilator (into the 3 o'clock, 6 o'clock, and 9 o'clock positions) as you squeeze. After you relax, see if you can press your dilator a little further, taking up the space you just created with your stretch. Repeat three times at each position, or at any place along your "smile" where you feel soreness and tightness.

PROGRESS: Progress to the next size dilator when you feel ready. The timetable for progression will vary greatly from person to person, depending on how often you stretch with your dilators and how tight your muscles are at the beginning. Repeat all of the techniques just listed with each progressively larger dilator.

———————

Congratulations! You have achieved some amazing relaxation and elongation of your pelvic floor. This process takes time, but the incredible benefits in pain relief will be well worth your effort. Jessica's husband helped massage, stretch, and dilate Jessica's pelvic floor in a team effort. She showed him how, and he felt comfortable and needed!

Strengthening Exercises

Generally speaking, most physical therapists advocate stretching before strengthening when it comes to pelvic pain treatment. The primary problem in pelvic pain is chronic, painful shortening of the pelvic floor muscles, coupled with increased tone. Contracting a muscle shortens it, but it also brings wonderful blood flow and nourishment. For lots of people, muscles relax more fully once they are exercised. Exercise helps to release tone, too!

Quick Pelvic Floor Contractions

Three sessions of 10 repetitions (2-second contractions) comprise a good daily plan. These were fully covered in Chapter 3. Follow each strengthening session with a few deep inhalations with concurrent bulging/dropping of the pelvic floor. End with a relaxation exercise such as deep breathing.

Endurance Pelvic Floor Contractions

Three sets of 10 repetitions (10 seconds of holding, 10 seconds rest) would be a good regimen. These were fully covered in Chapter 3. Follow each strengthening session with a few deep inhalations with concurrent bulging/dropping of the pelvic floor.

Pelvic Floor Strengthening with the Pelvic Brace

Urinary incontinence often accompanies pelvic pain. Having a strong pelvic floor and transversus abdominus (which together comprise the pelvic brace) is needed for the treatment for stress incontinence and pelvic pain. A Reformer or mat Pilates exercise class, as presented in Chapter 6, would be ideal. Methods to find certified Pilates instructors are contained in Appendix III, page 248. The next two pages show some additional core strengthening exercises you can do with a physio-ball, if you have one.

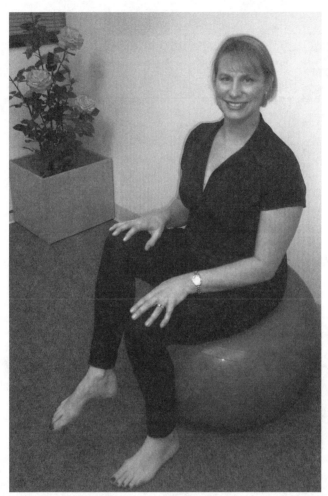

"Marching" with the pelvic brace on a physio-ball.

INSTRUCTIONS: While sitting on the physio-ball, engage the pelvic brace muscles by bringing your navel to your spine and squeezing your pelvic floor up. Hold these muscles. Keeping your hips level, raise one foot up as shown. Then lift the other foot. Strive to keep your balance by holding pelvic brace for 10 repetitions on each leg. To finish, breath in, and allow your pelvic floor to bulge or drop downward (toward your toes) as the air fills your trunk.

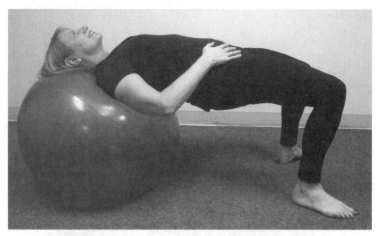

"Bridging" with the pelvic brace on a physio-ball.

INSTRUCTIONS: Assume the position pictured above on the physio-ball. Engage the pelvic brace muscles by bringing your navel to your spine and squeezing your pelvic floor up. Hold for 10 seconds, not allowing your pelvis to drop. Roll back a little to rest your core, and repeat 10 times. To finish, breath in, and allow your pelvic floor to bulge or drop downward (toward your toes) as the air fills your trunk.

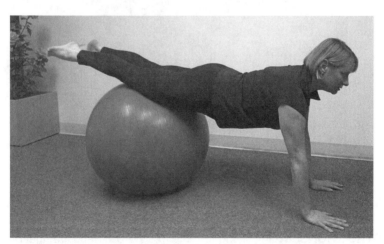

"Plank" exercise with the pelvic brace on a physio-ball.

INSTRUCTIONS: Assume the position pictured above on the physio-ball. Engage the pelvic brace muscles by bringing your navel to your spine and squeezing your pelvic floor. Hold for 10 seconds, not allowing your pelvis or shoulder blades to drop down. Roll back a little to rest your core, and repeat 10 times. To finish, breath in, and allow your pelvic floor to bulge or drop downward (toward your toes) as the air fills your trunk.

Behavioral Tips

There is a lot more you can do to manage and overcome your pelvic floor pain and sexual issues. In the following sections we provide brief descriptions of some helpful tips.

Before Sex

There is nothing more soothing to your body and to your pelvic floor muscles than a warm bath. Avoid perfumed soaps and bubble baths. You can perform your external and internal massage and stretching techniques in the bath, with or without your dilators. Using your larger vaginal dilator is a good precursor before sexual intercourse. Urinate before intercourse.

Tantric Sex

Sexual intercourse does not always have to involve a lot of (painful) action. The ancient practice of tantric sex allows a couple to have intercourse with a minimum of movement. First, relax your pelvic floor muscles by letting them drop and bulge with inhalation as you have learned. Second, teach your man how to slowly enter your vagina, coordinating his advance with your relaxed inhalations and pelvic floor dropping/bulging. It may take several deep breaths before he fully penetrates. In tantric sex, he stops moving and focuses on his sensual stimulation in connection with holding himself back. This gives your muscles time to stretch and relax, and it greatly lessens your worry over painful thrusting. Most men with partners who suffer from pelvic pain are usually quite willing to participate this way, especially if they know they are making the experience less painful for their partners.

After Sex

Urinate after sexual intercourse. Make a "condom popsicle" by filling a condom with water and freezing it ahead of time. Wrap a thin dishtowel around it and press it up against your perineum for ten minutes to help reduce post-intercourse soreness and inflammation. Try to keep your pelvic floor muscles relaxed by bulging and dropping with your deep inhalations.

Aerobic Exercise

Thirty to forty-five minutes of aerobic exercise per day is a natural stress reliever, and the associated endorphin release is a natural painkiller. Walking and swimming are wonderful choices.

Relieving Stress

There is a strong relationship between the mind and the body. Modern medicine no longer balks at this concept as it once did. The way we think influences how we feel. Catastrophic thoughts, such as "I am going to have this pain forever," can indeed perpetuate the pain. Positive thinking, such as "I am a little better today because I can sit longer and more comfortably," facilitates recovery. Stay positive and avoid the negative conversations you may be having with yourself.

Let your "gratitude attitude" shine forth, as coined by the book and movie *The Secret*, by Rhonda Byrne (2006). Visualize a pain-free life, be consistent with your massage and exercises, and you will achieve the life you want to lead. Guided visualizations to clear your head of stressful thoughts are described in Chapter 9 on page 232. Visualize your soft, elastic, long, and happy pelvic floor muscles, and soon that's what you'll have!

In this chapter, you have been given a veritable buffet of ways to relax, massage, stretch, strengthen, tone, and strengthen the pelvic floor and surrounding muscles. How often you perform each of these exercises will depend on *you*—how you are feeling and how much time you have to devote. You probably won't be able to do everything every day. Most women prefer to massage their muscles before stretching them. You must experiment with all the different techniques and exercises to see what works best for you. Just make it a priority in your life!

We wish we could devote 200 pages to the assessment and treatment of pelvic floor pain. We have provided you with a chapter full of useful information and helpful treatment techniques, but this topic really warrants its own book. We recommend two excellent books to augment this chapter, both written by physical therapists practicing in New York City: *Heal Pelvic Pain: A Proven Stretching, Strengthening, and Nutrition Program for Relieving Pain, Incontinence, IBS, and Other Symptoms Without Surgery*, by Amy Stein, MPT, which we mentioned earlier in this chapter, and *Ending Female Pain: A Woman's Manual, the Ultimate Self-Help Guide for Women Suffering from Chronic Pelvic and Sexual Pain* by Isa Herrera, MSPT, CSCS (see Appendix III, page 250).

A condensed review of this chapter follows. Photocopy it and keep it in your bedroom. Rely on this physical therapy home program, and soon you will be sending your pelvic pain on a one-way trip → Out of your life for good!

YOUR HOME PROGRAM FOR PELVIC PAIN AND SEXUAL ISSUES

1. **Relaxing and Stretching Your Pelvic Floor Muscles (~5 minutes total time)**
   - Diaphragmatic breathing to relieve tension: twice
   - Add bulging/dropping your pelvic floor muscles with inhalation: twice
   - Add pelvic floor stretches with breathing in and bulging/dropping your pelvic floor:
     ◦ Squatting" on Your Back": Hold ~1 minute
     ◦ Child's Pose: Hold ~1 minute
     ◦ Frog Squat: Hold ~1 minute

2. **Stretching Exercises for Muscles Surrounding the Pelvis (~1 minute each)**

Lying on your back:	• Pretzel stretch
	• Hamstring stretch
	• Figure 4 stretch
On your tummy:	• Sphinx
Half-sitting on chair:	• Side stretch while dropping hip
Standing with one leg on chair:	• Hip Flexor stretch

3. **External Self-Massage (~5 minutes total time, ideally with/after a bath)**

Sit on physio-ball:	• "Bounce" and "Gyrate"
Sit on soft → hard small balls:	• Inside of sit bones (right and left) and in middle of pelvic floor
Backnobber® massage:	• To pelvic floor (standing with one foot on chair)
	• To upper/lower back & hamstrings

Jacknobber® massage:

- To buttocks, inner thighs, gluteals, piriformis, waist

Middle finger on outside of pelvic floor:

- "Snowflake" massage

4. Internal Self-Massage
(~5 minutes total time, ideally with/after a bath)

Thumb massage:
- Clock massage stretch at 3, 6, and 9 o'clock
- Smile massage sweeping between 3 o'clock and 9 o'clock
- Contract pelvic floor around thumb, while thumb is pressing on tender points to deactivate them

Vaginal dilators:
- Gradually increase from smallest to largest
- Clock massage: 3, 6, and 9 o'clock with dilator
- Smile massage sweeping between 3 o'clock and 9 o'clock
- Contract pelvic floor with dilator in center of vagina
- Contract pelvic floor with dilator pressing on tender points to deactivate them

5. Strengthening Exercises
- Quick pelvic floor contractions: 10 repetitions of 2-second contractions, 3 times a day.
- Endurance pelvic floor contractions: 10 repetitions of 10-second contractions, 3 times a day
- Physio-ball exercises with pelvic brace: 10 each, once a day
  - Marching
  - Bridge
  - Plank

6. Behavioral Tips
- Before sex: Bathe, breathe and relax, self-massage, stretch, urinate
- Tantric sex
- After sex: Urinate, use cold compress, breathe and relax
- General aerobic exercise: ~30 to 45 minutes per day

7. Relieving Stress
(throughout the day)
- Positive thinking
- "Gratitude attitude"

"Promise me you'll always remember: You're braver than you believe, stronger than you seem, and smarter than you think."
—Christopher Robin to Pooh, A. A. Milne

 **9 Moving from Depression to Joy**

"THE VACATIONLESS": MEET YVONNE

At age 62, I had the biggest jolt of my life: My husband of 38 years died unexpectedly. He was the first and only love of my life. He had recently retired, and we had planned the celebration trip of a lifetime. I was devastated and spent the better part of a year in depression, mourning my loss.

Although the trip would never be the same without my beloved Walter, my family encouraged me to take it anyway, with my good friend Marie, also a widow. It was the best thing I could have done. When I returned home, my family barely recognized me. Though I still missed my husband dearly, I had regained some of my zest for life.

Marie and I began planning our next adventure. Each week we met for lunch at a different restaurant that served traditional food from a country we thought we might visit. We each came armed with brochures and research on different destinations. After months of information gathering, we finally narrowed it down: three weeks in Australia! The Outback fascinated us, and we could hardly wait to see the Great Barrier Reef.

Unfortunately, one pivotal day on the golf course spoiled all of my wonderful travel plans. I have what I call a sensitive bladder, but the pads I wear are super absorbent, so I always feel confident. My bladder gets worse in times of stress. That was definitely true after Walter died, when I found myself changing my pads all the time and sleeping in diapers.

There I was, on the golf course about to tee-off, when I realized I had to go to the bathroom right away! The only restroom was at the clubhouse, hundreds of yards away. I didn't know what to do and found myself urinating before I could decide. I stood unmoving as my golf pants became wet.

I was playing with some ladies I knew from the club, but they were not close friends. They tried not to make a big scene out of it, and one graciously offered me her golf sweater to wrap around my waist. I considered trying to play on, but I was starting to smell. I finally gave in to the shame, excused myself from our game, and walked back to my car, avoiding the clubhouse and any people along the way.

At home, I cried in the shower while thoughts of dread darted through my mind. I had noticed my urges getting stronger over the last several months, but nothing like this, when my pad proved useless. I could never let that happen again. What about my trip? While Marie and I were traveling in the Australian bush, we would often be miles from the next modern bathroom! Traveling in diapers was my only choice.

Resolved to my grim situation, I tried to focus on the positive and redirected my energy toward planning my trip. Our last lunch before the trip was at a great Australian bistro we had come to enjoy. Marie handed me a typed itinerary that detailed all of our flight reservations and ground transport information. At the bottom was a list of the Transportation Security Administration (TSA) guidelines and baggage restrictions. It was at that point that I froze.

There was no way I would be able to meet the baggage requirements. My diapers alone took up one huge suitcase, because I used two diapers during the day and one at night. Over the course of three weeks I would need 63 bulky diapers, and I certainly couldn't count on buying them in the Australian Outback!

Our trip was only two weeks away, yet I knew I couldn't go. I had to call Marie. It was one of the saddest things I ever did. I didn't reveal the real reason for my last-minute change of heart, but I suggested alternatives. When I mentioned going on a cruise instead, Marie said adamantly, "I am not going on an old lady cruise!" In truth, I felt the same, but I didn't know what else to say. I ended up canceling my part of the trip and I paid dearly for it. Marie and I no longer speak.

Today I spend most of my time at home, watching TV and dozing between shows. Often, I don't bother getting dressed. I don't go out much for fear of another accident, like the one I had at the club. My family says I'm depressed, and I must admit there are days when I feel I have nothing to live for.

Imagine the profound emptiness Yvonne must feel. She was hit by the shock of her husband's early death and then crippled by her own physical and psychological demons. Her incontinence has caused her to become a virtual shut-in, and her depression has left her sluggish, with no desire to do anything. She has been on an emotional rollercoaster built up by hope and joy and then destroyed by defeat and failure.

We regret to say that Yvonne's problem is not rare. The combination of urinary incontinence and depression is an actual medical syndrome. According to a large Canadian study, these conditions frequently occur together, and their combined impact exceeds the impact of either condition alone (Vigood & Stewart, 2006).

Yvonne has always had an incontinence issue; the question is, did she always have a depression issue? Which came first? Was her husband's death the catalyst that spurred her depression, or did the depression simply become more intense after he died? Her incontinence became more acute after his death, resulting in Yvonne using diapers to shield her accidents. Was it her grief over his death that caused that progression, or did her incontinence exacerbate her depressive state? The answers to these questions are not known.

Although Yvonne seemed to regain her sparkle by planning trips, her urge urinary incontinence forced her to withdraw, and she cycled back into a depressive state. Not having control of one's own life and bodily functions is depressing. Feeling shackled by both her incontinence and her depression, Yvonne has shunned the outside world and chosen a life of isolation, which is a leading contributing factor to depression in women.

Women suffering from this double syndrome often find themselves in a hole with no way out. We are here—with a rope—and we beg you to try to see the light. This chapter can be a new beginning for you.

We will start with some basic education about depression before we delve into the dual syndrome of incontinence and depression. Although neither of us is a psychologist, we will share some insight into this disorder and give you some tools and resources to begin the mending process. Research has shown that the more people educate themselves on their illnesses, the greater their chances of regaining health. Trust yourself to become the person you deserve to be. Carpe diem: Seize the day!

WHAT IS DEPRESSION?

Diagnosing incontinence is relatively simple, because the symptoms are obvious. Depression, on the other hand, is not as cut and dried. If you have times of sadness or have had a patch of blues after giving birth, are you clinically depressed? If you feel achy and tired all the time, are you depressed, or are you just coming down with the flu? Let's begin our education with some background on depression.

Depression affects nearly 20 million Americans each year, many of whom have a concurrent condition, such as diabetes, incontinence, cancer, or stroke. Forty to sixty-five percent of heart attack survivors also develop depression (National Institute of Mental Health, n.d.). The U.S. Department of Health and Human Services (2008) provided the following facts about depression. Women are twice as likely to be depressed as men. Women of all ages, ethnic origins, and socioeconomic backgrounds are diagnosed with clinical depression every day. Depression is the *Number One* cause of disability in women. Married women experience depression at greater rates than single women, and one group in which depression is prevalent are stay-at-home moms with small children. Sixty percent of people who commit suicide had major depression, and although more men than women kill themselves each year in the United States, women attempt suicide twice as often as men.

Clinical/Major Depression Versus "The Blues"

Many of us have had days when we have felt low, or periods of sadness due to a life-changing event in our lives, such as the death of a loved one. Those melancholy emotions are a normal part of being human. However, major depression occurs when those feelings continue and begin to affect one's life on a daily basis, over a longer period of time. Major depression is an all-encompassing feeling of despondency that can influence a person's job, family life, appetite, sleeping habits, and general health.

Depression and its symptoms are different for every sufferer. Some women have described a feeling of profound doom and paralyzing sadness, whereas others don't feel sad at all—just lethargic and unmotivated to do much of anything.

SIGNS OF DEPRESSION

- Loss of energy or fatigued for no obvious reason
- Feelings of emptiness or hopelessness
- Loss of sexual desire
- Sleeping too much or too little
- No appetite or overeating, resulting in marked weight loss or weight gain

- Lack of desire to do anything, including basic tasks or favorite activities
- Feelings of anger
- Overwhelming sadness
- Inability to concentrate, focus, remember, or make decisions
- Thoughts of suicide or injuring oneself

As we mentioned earlier, determining whether you are incontinent is easy, but detecting depression can be more complex. Depression is hard to self-diagnose. Depressed women become conditioned to their low feelings and begin to believe they are normal. The well-known analogy of a boiling frog is a perfect example of this. If you put a live frog in boiling water, it will jump out. However, if you put that same frog in cool water and slowly turn up the heat, the frog, unaware of the impending danger, will eventually cook to death. The same general principle applies to humans. We may not react to gradual changes that occur over time, regardless of their significance. For this reason, a friend or relative may be the first to notice and point out your depressed state. Although news like this is hard to hear, resist the temptation to ignore it. Instead, trust others close to you and take steps toward feeling good again.

Later in this chapter, we discuss the causes of depression, offer self-testing tools, and give suggestions to help improve your outlook on life. Now, however, we want to discuss the concurrent conditions of incontinence and depression, and how this association came to be.

ACKNOWLEDGING THE CONNECTION
BETWEEN INCONTINENCE AND DEPRESSION

Although the cliché "Which came first, the chicken or the egg?" has been used many times before, it is ever so fitting for this subject. One might guess that anyone with severe incontinence would be depressed. This makes sense, because incontinence is an emotionally challenging and life-altering condition; however, that hypothesis is not necessarily true. Not all women suffering with urinary incontinence are clinically depressed. Learning that was *not* the biggest surprise we found when researching this topic. Instead, we were dumbfounded to learn that *depression* is often the *first* illness, followed by incontinence—which once again begs the classic question, "Which came first . . . ?"

Researchers have spent decades studying the correlation between urinary incontinence and depression. Although there are still no definitive answers, the theories are compelling. Regardless of the reason behind the connection, it most certainly exists. The following summary of current research may help you gain a better understanding of the relationship between incontinence and depression, and why they coincide in your life.

A Chemical Connection

An imbalance in certain chemicals in the brain, called *neurotransmitters*, may cause depression. These neurotransmitters are responsible for sending messages back and forth within the brain to help with bodily functions as well as to regulate behaviors such as mood, sexual desire, appetite, sleep, and memory. *Serotonin* is one of these neurotransmitters. Some researchers believe that a serotonin imbalance in the brain couples incontinence with depression.

Serotonin also affects bladder function. Connection made! "Serotonin inhibits the voiding reflex and has a role in increasing urethral tone" (Bent, Cundiff, & Swift, 2007, p. 315). An article published in the *Journal of Urology* made the following claim:

> Serotonergic neuronal systems have been implicated in anxiety and depression. Because descending serotonin pathways from the brain stem inhibit bladder contractions, it is postulated that depression associated with altered serotonin function may predispose [one] to urge incontinence. An association between depression and idiopathic urge incontinence is demonstrated. (Zorn et al., 1999, p. 82)

These researchers believe that the depression–incontinence association may be due to altered serotonin function and may help explain the effectiveness of serontonergic-based antidepressants in the treatment of urge incontinence.

In a more recent study, documented in the *American Journal of Obstetrics and Gynecology*, researchers investigated the causal link between depression and incontinence. Data gathered and analyzed over a period of six years was part of an ongoing project called the Health and Retirement Study. The financial and physical health of recent retirees in 70,000 American households was assessed. The researchers examined women who entered the study with depression and screened them for urinary incontinence over the course of the study. Conversely, women presenting with urinary incontinence at baseline were queried to see whether depression was reported at follow-up (Melville et al., 2009).

The results showed that, out of 5,820 women (in their mid to late fifties) who reported depression at the start of the study, twenty-one percent developed urinary incontinence; however, *none* of the women with urinary incontinence developed depression (Melville et al., 2009). Thus, major depression was a predictor for the initial development of incontinence; incontinence was not a predictor for depression. Although the researchers did not have enough data to pin the blame on chemical imbalance, they suggested it as a possible cause for the onset of incontinence.

Still a Mystery . . .

Although it is widely speculated that insufficient serotonin levels play a significant role in depression, and perhaps in urge incontinence, no one knows for sure. We have no test that can measure the serotonin level in a living brain. As a result, no studies can prove that brain levels of neurotransmitters are deficient when depression develops. We can, however, measure serotonin in the blood, and depressed women generally have lower blood serotonin levels. Unfortunately, the conundrum endures, because doctors are unsure whether the depression caused the serotonin levels to drop or the low serotonin levels caused the depression.

NOTE: If you are currently taking medication for either urinary incontinence or depression and have experienced the other condition as well, share this information with your doctor. He or she may be able to adjust your dosage or change your prescription to counter any unwanted side effects. Your local pharmacist can also be a fantastic ally to help educate you about drug interactions.

Impact on Quality of Life

Urinary incontinence interferes with the quality of one's life. The degree to which it interferes may vary, depending on the severity of the incontinence as well as the current lifestyle expectations of the incontinent woman. A study of large populations of incontinent women revealed that they were nearly twice as likely as continent women to have major depression (Vigod & Stewart, 2006). Women suffering from the double syndrome were often absent from work and had more frequent doctor visits. Also, "Women with urinary incontinence who were 18–44 had the highest prevalence of depression, almost three times that of women age 45 or older" (Vigod & Stewart, 2006, p. 150). Furthermore, young continent women with multiple chronic conditions were generally less depressed than young incontinent women, leading the researchers to believe there is something unique and possibly more profoundly disruptive about life with urinary incontinence.

Isolation

Regardless of age, many incontinent women become reclusive, and isolation is their safety net. Incontinence can generate feelings of embarrassment, doom, and inadequacy; depression shares many of these same traits. Socializing with friends, joining clubs, or leaving the house to do simple tasks (e.g., grocery shopping) is not easy for a depressed, incontinent woman. Many women with acute urge incontinence live in constant fear of accidents, often requiring unrelenting bathroom mapping. They feel it is safer and simpler to just stay home.

Lack of Physical Activity

An American study of 3,364 women revealed that "85.3% of women surveyed with severe incontinence consider their problem being a chief obstacle to physical exercise, compared to the 64.5% of women with average incontinence" (Brown & Miller, 2001, p. 373–378). Lack of activity can result in boredom, fatigue, and an overall sense of the blues. In addition, the absence of exercise can perpetuate weight gain and put a woman at risk for such medical conditions as high blood pressure, osteoporosis, and heart disease.

Decrease in Sex Life

Sexual dysfunction is often found in women with urinary incontinence, resulting in lack of interest, stimulation, orgasm, and overall satisfaction. Some women with certain types of incontinence, such as nocturnal enuresis (bedwetting), avoid sex altogether. One does not feel very sexy wearing bulky pads or diapers to bed. According to an article in the *Cleveland Clinic Journal of Medicine*, "In essence, a woman's perception of her own sexuality is jeopardized, leading to significant inhibition" (Barber et al., 2005, p. 229). Having sexual relations involves too much rigamarole for many women with nocturnal enuresis. It involves disposing of a wet pad, cleaning, placing a towel underneath, and then recleaning, and repadding afterward. Odor and partners' reactions play big roles, leading to embarrassment and psychological distress for women. Lack of sexual desire is a possible sign of depression as well.

Financial Burden

The extra cost of management materials, such as pads and diapers, can create a huge financial burden. Not only are incontinent patients facing the humiliation, alienation, and depression their problem inherently brings, but they also might be going into debt because of it.

Whether the connection between incontinence and depression is chemical, environmental, or cause and effect from one to the other, the link *is* there. Your incontinence puts you at risk for depression, and vice versa; therefore, we strongly recommend that you be screened for both conditions.

Various self-screening tests for depression are available on the Internet. These confidential screenings can be done in the privacy of your own home, so you can assess yourself for possible depression. Most will rank your answers to a series of questions and give you a numeric score, thereby rating the severity of your depression. These tools can be very empowering because they are often the first step in seeking help. After taking one of these tests, you will have compelling data to share with your physician, so you can begin a treatment program.

The good news is that the success rate of treating women with depression is extremely high. We have included websites for self-testing depression and related resources in Appendix III (page 248). Select one and complete a test today.

If you are wondering how you got here in the first place, let's look at the causes of depression. First, understand that depression is *real*. It is not a personality or character flaw. It is not confined to people who had difficult childhoods, and it is not a "made-up" condition. These inaccurate social stigmas only make people with depression more insecure about the authenticity of their illness. If you are depressed, you are in good company. Surprisingly, some of the most famous people in history have been clinically depressed, including Abraham Lincoln, Mark Twain, Marilyn Monroe, and Beethoven. You are also among the millions of people struggling with depression everyday. Let's try to find out why.

Causes of Depression

Genetics

Can a person be genetically predisposed to depression? Some researchers believe that major depression can indeed be genetic and run in families. In fact, a recent analysis of fifty-four studies suggested just that: "People with a short variation of the serotonin transporter (5-HTTLPR) gene are more likely to become depressed when faced with certain stressful life events than their counterparts who have the longer variation" (Karg et al., 2011, p. 444–445).

Chemical Imbalance

We covered the link between brain chemicals and depression earlier in this chapter, and scientists continue to conduct research to help validate their theories. Pharmaceutical products for incontinence, depression, or other ailments should be discussed with your treating doctor to investigate whether certain drugs or drug combinations are negatively affecting your overall health and well-being.

Hormonal Factors

Hormonal factors include menstrual cycles; pregnancy; and the postpartum, perimenopause, and menopause phases. All of these reproductive stages affect your natural hormone balance and, depending on the individual, these hormonal disruptions can produce adverse effects.

Environmental Factors

Stress at work, stress at home, the strain of caring for an elderly parent, or the burdens of single parenthood can lead to depression. A life-altering event, such as a death or divorce, also can spawn such feelings.

Medical Illness

A stroke, heart attack, cancer, or other debilitating disease can be a precursor to depression.

BECOMING WHOLE AGAIN

The most important first step you can make toward getting this syndrome under control is to talk with your doctor. Share with him or her that you are experiencing *both* depression and incontinence. If the doctor is your OB/GYN or general/family practitioner, bring your depression screening quiz and share your results. If he or she is your psychiatrist, bring your incontinence self-assessment, found in Appendix I, page 243. Encourage your doctors to treat the "whole" you.

Discuss with your doctor any medications you are currently taking and their possible adverse side effects. Investigate whether there are medications available to help get you on a faster track toward recovery and get you feeling good again. Many antidepressants and mood stabilizers have been lifesavers for depressed patients, helping with such problems as mood swings, lack of motivation, anxiety, and suicidal thoughts.

NOTE: If you have stopped taking your regular prescriptions during pregnancy, talk to your doctor about beginning them again. Certain medications may be OK to use while breastfeeding, but check with your doctor first.

If urinary incontinence *is* the primary source of your depression, this book can help end your incontinence and give you hope for ending your depression as well. As you have learned earlier in this book, controlling your urinary incontinence takes work. Continue to do the exercises you learned in Chapters 3 and 5. If you have fallen off the exercise wagon, hop back on. Don't get overwhelmed with the entire eight-week program; take it one day at a time. As you slowly bring the pelvic floor exercises and urge suppression techniques into your routine, celebrate with something special. Create a reward system for yourself that will motivate you to persevere as you retrain your bladder. Make the rewards something worthwhile that you really enjoy—a special meal, a manicure, or a new pair of shoes, for example.

If you have been diagnosed with depression and are in the initial stages of treatment, you won't become better overnight. Overcoming sad emotions takes time. In the next section we suggest a few ways to create some sunshine in an otherwise dim room.

Tips for Feeling Happier

Watch a Funny Movie

Watch your favorite type of comedy, be it slapstick or romantic. Rent them by the dozens if you can. Over 25 years ago, Dr. Norman Cousins wrote the book *Anatomy of an Illness as Perceived by the Patient* (1981). After he was diagnosed with a debilitating illness and given little hope for recovery, he began watching Marx Brothers movies daily. Cousins believes he was able to laugh his way to recovery. A lifetime fitness advocate, he believed that human emotions are the key to overall health and well-being. An avid runner, Cousins (1981) said that laughter was like "inner jogging."

We do understand that although side-splitting laughter may be therapeutic to someone with depression, it can be detrimental to someone with incontinence. In this case, the fight against depression dominates. Watch the movies at home and dress comfortably. At this point, the benefit of the laughter will outweigh any accidents. As you continue to improve your pelvic floor strength, laughing your guts out will no longer be a problem.

Exercise

Start with short walks and work your way up to more active exercise. The fresh air, sunlight, and endorphins generated by the physical activity will do wonders for your mood. Swimming and cycling are wonderful low-impact aerobic choices.

Enjoy Lunch with a Friend

For someone suffering from depression, a social event, even with one close friend, can be a daunting proposition. You may have to push yourself into an uncomfortable zone. However, getting out and socializing again will remind you of happier times, and you will reap the rewards.

Avoid Starchy and Sugary Foods

Comfort foods, which often are full of starch and/or sugar, can be detrimental to certain individuals suffering from depression. Some studies show that high-fat, high-sugar diets reduce the effectiveness of certain chemicals in the brain. In fact, according to Fernando Gómez-Pinilla, UCLA professor of neurology and physiological science, junk food and fast food negatively affect the brain's synapses. Gómez-Pinilla, who has spent years studying the effects of food on the brain, shares that while foods rich in omega-3 fatty acids and folic acids can help increase brain function, the reverse is also true. Diets deficient in these important nutrients have been associated with increased risk of several mental disorders, including depression.

Revisit a Favorite Place or Activity

Conjure up a favorite place or activity that you haven't experienced in years. Go there mentally (i.e., imagine being there) or physically to lift your mood and renew your carefree attitude.

Do Yoga

If you have never done yoga, you are in for a treat. Many city park programs, YMCAs, local gyms, or senior centers offer yoga. The mind–body experience you will receive is invigorating.

Get a Massage

The touch of massage can alleviate stress and renew your spirit. Treat yourself. It is very hard to be angry while receiving a soothing massage.

Meditate

Meditation or visualization can be very healing. Letting go of worries and stress and focusing on the moment can be empowering. The following "Mirrored Hallway" technique, adapted from Hererra (2009), is a wonderful guided visualization you can try for relaxation.

The "Mirrored Hallway" Visualization

Close your eyes, take five slow relaxing breaths, and don't think about the past or the future. Imagine yourself entering a narrow 8-foot hallway. You see a door on the other end. You notice that there are floor-to-ceiling mirrors on both long walls.

On your *left*, you see yourself and your situation, and your reflection shows your pain, your anxiety, your negative outlook, and anything in your life you wish to overcome.

On your *right*, the mirror shows the exact opposite of you. You see yourself as pain-free, happy, fulfilled, and able to overcome anything that life puts in your path. Dwell on this image and absorb it.

You notice a large shepherd's staff propped in the left corner. You pick it up, and you smash the mirror on the left with one forceful blow, as you tell yourself you will *not* allow those reflections to exist any longer.

Gaze and smile at the reflection at the right as you walk toward the door and through it, taking the best of you into the world and continuing your journey as a pain-free person.

The next section is your home program, a cheat sheet of sorts, to help guide you toward a happier you. Use it in good health and know we are pulling for you!

YOUR HOME PROGRAM TO REGAIN THE JOY IN YOUR LIFE

■ **Visit Your Physician with Complete Disclosure**. Bring your incontinence self-assessment from Appendix I (page 243) and a depression self-test from Appendix III (page 248) in order to share all of your ongoing symptoms with your physician. Discuss all medications you are taking (including any potential drug interactions), and be open minded about additional treatment.

- **Maintain Your Pelvic Floor Health**. Follow the comprehensive home programs outlined in Chapters 3 and 5. If you have slacked off from doing your exercises, begin again. Create a reward system to help keep you motivated. Taking control of your bladder will make you feel more in control of your life, diminishing your feelings of depression.

- **Incorporate Your Pelvic Brace Into Your Daily Life**. Remember to contract your pelvic brace during coughing, sneezing, nose blowing, lifting, stair climbing, and any strenuous activity that adds pressure to your bladder and pelvic floor.

- **Create Joy Again in Your Life**. Watch a funny movie, enjoy lunch with a friend, or go out for an evening. Revisit a favorite place or participate in a favorite game or activity. Remind yourself of what happy feels like!

- **Exercise Regularly and with Low Impact**. Get daily aerobic exercise, even if you begin with slow, short walks. Enjoy the positive "rush" from exercise-induced endorphins.

- **Find Inner Peace**. Meditate, go to church, or do yoga. Give yourself some quiet time to breathe, relax, and focus on a positive you.

- **Plan a Special Event**. Give yourself something to look forward to, such as a party or a vacation.

Acknowledging your dual hurdles of incontinence and depression is a heroic leap. We hope that the information we shared in this chapter helps you to better understand this complicated connection. New facets of this syndrome are still being uncovered, so keep abreast of new information as it becomes available. Arm yourself with the knowledge to take this on and *win*!

Urinary incontinence with major depression is highly prevalent in women, and both conditions require treatment. We hope to draw attention to this topic and empower women to approach their doctors with knowledge and confidence. Creating more awareness of the relationship between these two conditions will establish earlier diagnoses and treatment, ultimately improving the quality of life of millions of women. Being in control of our bodies and our circumstances are key ingredients to physical and mental health.

> "The will to win, the desire to succeed, the urge to reach your full potential . . . these are the keys that will unlock the door to personal excellence."
> —Confucius

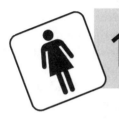

10 How Dry I Am . . . How Wet I'll Be . . . If I Don't Find . . . THE BATHROOM KEY

How dry I am; how wet I'll be
If I don't find the bathroom key
I found the key; I found the door
But it's too late; it's on the floor!

Do you know this folk song? This tune was sung in Kathryn's childhood home, whenever one of her five family members needed to use an occupied bathroom. After several polite requests and knocks, this song was howled through the door crack as the final threat, along with some heavy banging! It was an effective ritual to eject the offending "bathroom hog" when one just couldn't *wait*!

This book was written at the urgency (and we do mean that literally) of thousands of patients who couldn't wait to get rid of their bladder control issues, and the millions of others who remain without help. Not a day passes without at least one patient telling Kathryn, "No one *knows* about physical therapy for *this*! You should write a book!" Of course, when Kim (as Kathryn's patient) said *she* was going to do it, they decided to join forces, and the idea of *The Bathroom Key* was conceived.

We are honored to have our book in your hands. You have found the *key*, and now we want you to find the *door*—to the right medical professional—if you desire help beyond the pages of this book.

For some people, this book alone is enough to eliminate your bladder leakage, and it was written for you. We have sailed into every dock on the waterfront, so to speak: stress and urge urinary incontinence, urgency, frequency, nocturia, nocturnal enuresis, urinary tract infections, organ prolapse, chronic pelvic pain, and depression with incontinence. You know more about Dr. Arnold Kegel and Joseph Pilates than most graduating medical students.

For other readers, this book's greatest value is to make you aware of the powerful effectiveness of physical therapy for your incontinence, prolapse, or pelvic pain. Most insurance plans will cover individualized, one-on-one physical therapy treatment (including surface electromyographic biofeedback). In this chapter, we *prepare* and *teach* you how to find the right professionals, what to say to those professionals, and what to bring with you—so that your doctor, physical therapist, or Pilates instructor will tend to *your* specific needs. The last line of the folk song is wrong; it's *never* too late!

YOUR SELF-ASSESSMENT QUESTIONNAIRE

It's always motivational to know you are improving. Did you complete the self-assessment questionnaire in Appendix I, page 243, when you began reading this book, back in Chapter 1? Well, it's time to take it again and assess your progress. The following short form will be quite inspirational to see objective evidence of your improvement (with a numeric score), and you should compare it with your previous score or scores. However, spending less money on pads is a pretty objective indicator of success, too!

This form will also help your clinicians. Kathryn created this form for this book because the only available questionnaires had been developed for research purposes and lacked good quantification of symptoms. The older forms rely heavily on the perceptions and subjective knowledge of the person completing them. For example, how could you rate your urinary frequency as "a little," "moderate," or "a lot," if you have no idea what *normal frequency* is? You will help your clinician so much more by showing her that you answered "b" to Question 4, for example. That would inform her that you urinate about every two hours, and she would know you have a moderate frequency problem.

KASSAI SELF-ASSESSMENT FOR URINARY CONTROL

1. **In the past 6 months have you ever accidentally leaked urine when you didn't want to—even a minor amount?**
    1 YES   0 NO → SKIP questions 2 and 3.

2. **What causes you to have leakage of urine?**
    CIRCLE (a), (b), OR (c)
    - **(a)** 3   PHYSICAL ACTIVITIY: Coughing, sneezing, laughing, nose blowing, lifting, squatting, standing up from a chair, stair climbing, walking, running, playing sports. ← **CIRCLE the activities.** *(Stress Urinary Incontinence)*
    - **(b)** 3   BEING ON THE WAY TO THE BATHROOM: Getting a strong urge to urinate that is too strong or comes on too soon. *(Urge Urinary Incontinence)*
    - **(c)** 6   BOTH (a) and (b) *(Mixed Urinary Incontinence)*

3. **Do you wear protective pads?**
    0 NO   YES → **CIRCLE:**   1 Liners   2 Pads   3 Diapers
    I wear a total of approximately:
    - **(a)** 1   7 or fewer products per WEEK.
    - **(b)** 2   8 to 14 products per WEEK.
    - **(c)** 3   15 to 21 products per WEEK.
    - **(d)** 4   22 or more products per WEEK.

4. **How often do you use the toilet to urinate during the day?**
    - **(a)** 0   About every three to four hours throughout the day *(No Frequency)*
    - **(b)** 1   About every two hours throughout the day *(Moderate Frequency)*
    - **(c)** 2   About every hour (or less) throughout the day *(Severe Frequency)*

5. **How many times do you get up from bed to use the bathroom each night?**
    - **(a)** 0   I sleep through the night. *(No Nocturia)*
    - **(b)** 1   I get up once to use the bathroom. *(Mild Nocturia)*
    - **(c)** 2   I get up twice to use the bathroom. *(Moderate Nocturia)*
    - **(d)** 3   I get up three or more times to use the bathroom. *(Severe Nocturia)*

6. **How have your bladder issues changed your life?**
   CIRCLE all that apply:

   (a) 0   I can do everything without any difficulty.

   (b) 1   I have some difficulty exercising, running, or doing sports.

   (c) 2   I have some difficulty doing household chores / shopping / running errands.

   (d) 2   I have trouble sitting through a movie or concert.

   (e) 2   I have trouble taking longer car trips.

   (f) 3   My bladder is controlling my life.

   (g) 3   I rarely socialize or take vacations out of town.

   (h) 3   I feel frustrated / nervous / depressed.

NAME:_____ DATE:_____

This form is reproducible WITHOUT written consent from Kathryn Kassai, PT.

<u>SCORE:</u>   */ 35 possible points*

How to Score the Kassai Self-Assessment Questionnaire for Urinary Control

Do you see the little numbers next to each answer? Simply add them together and write the total at the bottom of the form. A person with the worst possible case of urinary incontinence will receive a score of 35. The milder the symptoms, the lower the score will be.

Don't think that receiving a low (better) score "disqualifies" you from being treated medically. Every physical therapist on the planet would prefer to have the opportunity to treat patients with milder symptoms and prevent worsening of the incontinence. Conversely, if you are already in an assisted living home, it is not too late for you to seek help. The only normal requirements for physical therapy are that you are mentally and physically able to perform the exercises. Even if the incontinent person suffers from dementia, however, she can still benefit from physical therapy in the home as long as her caretaker receives the in-clinic education along with her.

Be as accurate as possible when describing your symptoms on this form. If you are uncertain how many times you get up to urinate at night or how many pads you actually use, fill out a copy of the Daily Voiding Diary (Appendix II, page 245) as described in Chapter 5. After that, filling out the Kassai Self-Assessment Questionnaire for Urinary Control will be a breeze! Bring both forms with you to your first visit with your doctor or physical therapist; they will offer a quick snapshot of the severity of your problem, so that an appropriate treatment plan can be devised just for *you*.

WHICH DOCTORS ASSESS URINARY INCONTINENCE?

Once upon a time, a "country doctor" took care of *all* of your medical needs. As recently as the 1950s, Dr. Arnold Kegel transitioned from being a thyroid surgeon to a gynecologist without doing a second, formal residency. However, that was before the body of medical knowledge grew so immense that formal specialization became unavoidable.

To find a physician to treat your incontinence issues, start with the doctor who knows you best, most likely your family physician or OB/GYN. If he or she feels you need to see a specializing physician, he or she will make the referral for you.

These are the types of physicians who have specialized training and thus will listen knowledgeably to your symptoms:

- **General practitioners, family practice physicians, and primary care physicians** treat patients of all ages.
- **Internists** focus on adult illness, injury, and prevention.
- **Obstetrician/gynecologists (OB/GYNs)** deliver babies and treat uterine, ovarian, vaginal, and female bladder issues.
- **Urologists** specialize in bladder issues for men and women.
- **Urogynecologists** have received dual training to treat female bladder and gynecological problems.

The National Association for Continence (http://www.nafc. org) maintains a database of medical providers who specialize in continence. When you supply your zip code, the site lists the nearby physicians.

> ## WHAT TO TAKE TO YOUR DOCTOR
>
> - A completed Daily Voiding Diary (page 245)
> - A completed Kassai Self-Assessment for Bladder Control (page 243)
> - A completed depression test or quiz you located with help from the information in Appendix III, Finding Physical Therapists and Other Resources (page 248)
> - A copy of this book, with any sections you wish to discuss flagged

Because you have read this book, you are now very well informed and prepared, so let it show! By completing the Daily Voiding Diary and the Kassai Self-Assessment for Bladder Control, you will impress your doctor with your thorough understanding of your symptoms. These forms will help you speak up and tell all. The detailed information you'll give your doctor will facilitate open and effective communication. After the physical examination, discuss with your doctor the nonsurgical, noninvasive, nonpharmacological approach of physical therapy and explain your desire to try it as first-line treatment for your incontinence. He or she will write a prescription (also called a *referral slip*) for physical therapy that you will give to your physical therapist.

FINDING A PHYSICAL THERAPIST WHO SPECIALIZES IN WOMEN'S HEALTH

Physical therapy clinics provide mainstream medical care and are located in most neighborhoods; however, most private clinics treat only orthopedic problems, and physical therapists who specialize in the pelvic floor are a bit more difficult to locate. Call local clinics and ask for a "physical therapist who specializes in pelvic floor rehabilitation or the treatment of incontinence." If they do not have this specialty, they will most likely know where to refer you. The pelvic floor physical therapist should gladly return your call and answer your questions. Her discussion of the services she provides should ring true with what you learned in this book. You may ask about her years of experience and the availability of SEMG biofeedback equipment at her clinic.

Turn to page 247 and consult the websites listed there. The American Physical Therapy Association (APTA), the Pelvic Rehab Institute, and the National Association for Continence (NAFC) maintain databases of qualified physical therapists specializing in Women's Health. By simply typing in your zip code, local physical therapists will appear. Of course, if you live near the zip code 90732, you can go to Kathryn's clinic (Praxis Physical Therapy) in San Pedro, California in Los Angeles County.

The only shame in having incontinence is not getting cured of it. We fervently hope that you are now self-confident about seeking the medical care you need—and do not feel awkward doing so. Whoopi Goldberg and Kris Kardashian Jenner have gone public with their urinary incontinence; however, it takes more than celebrity confessions to make this subject no longer taboo. It takes brave women such as yourself to speak up to your friends, family, and health care providers. Each woman who suffers with incontinence can do her part to diffuse the stigma and halt the progression of this distressing condition.

You have come out of the (water) closet. We are *so proud* of you for deciding to *do something* about your problem, instead of thinking of it as an inevitable result of aging or childbearing. We'd love to hear about your success story and how our book put you back in control. Please feel free to write to us at TheBathroomKey@aol.com, or visit our blog at www.TheBathroomKey.com and get updated educational information at our website.

Make the techniques presented in this book an integral part of how you live each day. You have stopped allowing your bladder to dominate your life, and we say "BRAVO!" Keep your determination *high* and your pad usage *low*. Before you know it, you will be bragging to all your friends and relatives about the embarrassing problem you *once had* and no longer do, encouraging them to follow your lead. Pay it forward!

We thank you for inviting us into your personal life, and we know you will not be disappointed with your transformation into the state of *dryness* and *freedom*. You deserve an active, exciting, independent life free of bladder issues. After all, a happy ending is really just the beginning.

Appendix I

Kassai Self-Assessment for Urinary Control

1. **In the past 6 months have you ever accidentally leaked urine when you didn't want to—even a minor amount?**
    1 YES   0 NO → SKIP questions 2 and 3.

2. **What causes you to have leakage of urine?**
    CIRCLE (a), (b), OR (c)
    - **(a)** 3 PHYSICAL ACTIVITIY: Coughing, sneezing, laughing, nose blowing, lifting, squatting, standing up from a chair, stair climbing, walking, running, playing sports. ← **CIRCLE the activities.**
      (Stress Urinary Incontinence)
    - **(b)** 3 BEING ON THE WAY TO THE BATHROOM: Getting a strong urge to urinate that is too strong or comes on too soon. *(Urge Urinary Incontinence)*
    - **(c)** 6 BOTH (a) and (b)   *(Mixed Urinary Incontinence)*

3. **Do you wear protective pads?**
    0 NO   YES → **CIRCLE:** 1 Liners   2 Pads   3 Diapers
    I wear a total of approximately:
    - **(a)** 1 7 or fewer products per WEEK.
    - **(b)** 2 8 to 14 products per WEEK.
    - **(c)** 3 15 to 21 products per WEEK.
    - **(d)** 4 22 or more products per WEEK.

4. **How often do you use the toilet to urinate during the day?**
    - **(a)** 0 About every three to four hours throughout the day
      (No Frequency)
    - **(b)** 1 About every two hours throughout the day
      (Moderate Frequency)
    - **(c)** 2 About every hour (or less) throughout the day
      (Severe Frequency)

5. **How many times do you get up from bed to use the bathroom each night?**
   - **(a)** 0   I sleep through the night. *(No Nocturia)*
   - **(b)** 1   I get up once to use the bathroom. *(Mild Nocturia)*
   - **(c)** 2   I get up twice to use the bathroom. *(Moderate Nocturia)*
   - **(d)** 3   I get up three or more times to use the bathroom. *(Severe Nocturia)*

6. **How have your bladder issues changed your life?**
   CIRCLE all that apply:
   - **(a)** 0   I can do everything without any difficulty.
   - **(b)** 1   I have some difficulty exercising, running, or doing sports.
   - **(c)** 2   I have some difficulty doing household chores / shopping / running errands.
   - **(d)** 2   I have trouble sitting through a movie or concert.
   - **(e)** 2   I have trouble taking longer car trips.
   - **(f)** 3   My bladder is controlling my life.
   - **(g)** 3   I rarely socialize or take vacations out of town.
   - **(h)** 3   I feel frustrated / nervous / depressed.

NAME:_____ DATE:_____

*SCORE:*_____ */ 35 possible points*

This form is reproducible WITHOUT written consent from Kathryn Kassai, PT.

Appendix II

Daily Voiding Diary

Column 1	Column 2	Column 3	Column 4	Column 5	Column 6
Time of Day	INTAKE: **TYPE of Food** **TYPE and AMOUNT of** **Beverages in Ounces**	Amount Voided in Toilet: • **In Ounces** OR • **In Seconds**	Amount of Leakage: **S / M / L** (small, medium, or large)	Was an Urge Present? **Yes / No**	**Which Activities** Caused Leakage?
Midnight					
1:00 a.m.					
2:00 a.m.					
3:00 a.m.					
4:00 a.m.					
5:00 a.m.					
6:00 a.m.					
7:00 a.m.					
8:00 a.m.					
9:00 a.m.					
10:00 a.m.					
11:00 a.m.					
Noon					
1:00 p.m.					
2:00 p.m.					
3:00 p.m.					
4:00 p.m.					
5:00 p.m.					
6:00 p.m.					
7:00 p.m.					
8:00 p.m.					
9:00 p.m.					
10:00 p.m.					
11:00 p.m.					

Body weight: _____lbs   TYPE and NUMBER of pads used today: _____

NAME: _____ DATE: _____

Appendix III

Finding Physical Therapists and Other Resources

HOW TO FIND PHYSICAL THERAPISTS WHO SPECIALIZE IN INCONTINENCE

Physical therapy is accepted mainstream medicine, and most health insurance plans cover it. Orthopedic clinics constitute the majority of private clinics in every neighborhood, however. Call local clinics and ask for a "physical therapist who specializes in pelvic floor rehabilitation or in the treatment of incontinence." If they don't have this specialty, they will most likely know where to refer you. The following organizations can help you locate a specialist:

- **Praxis Physical Therapy: http://www.praxisphysicaltherapy. com.** This is author Kathryn Kassai's website for her physical therapy clinic, located in San Pedro, California. It offers educational materials about urinary and fecal incontinence, Pilates, and other programs.
- **American Physical Therapy Association: http://www.womens healthapta.org/find-a-physical-therapist/index.cfm.** To find a physical therapist in your area who specializes in pelvic floor rehabilitation, go to the American Physical Therapy Association's website. By simply typing in your zip code, a local Women's Health physical therapist's name will appear, along with her specific areas of expertise.
- **Pelvic Rehab Institute: http://www.hermanwallace.com.** The Pelvic Rehab Institute provides expert training courses to physical therapists in pelvic floor/pelvic girdle dysfunction. The institute was founded by Holly Herman, DPT, and Kathe Wallace,

PT, and offers courses throughout the year on a variety of topics in this field. The institute maintains a practitioner directory of specializing physical therapists who have trained with them (including coauthor Kathryn Kassai, PT).

■ **National Association for Continence: http://www.nafc.org.** This database lists physical therapists and, when you enter your zip code, a nearby physical therapist may be listed.

HOW TO FIND PILATES INSTRUCTORS

Pilates classes are relatively easy to find, even in smaller cities. Start with your telephone book, because this will list all of the studios in your area. Also check with gyms, recreation centers, and YMCAs, because they, too, may offer mat and Reformer classes. Inquire whether the instructor has experience specific to urinary incontinence and pelvic floor rehabilitation.

Many Pilates certification programs offer directories of their graduates and studio locations. Try the following websites:

http://www.thepilatescenter.com
http://www.balancedbody.com
http://www.stottpilates.com
http://www.peakpilates.com

There also is a national organization that sets national guidelines and maintains instructor lists: **http://www.pilatesmethodalliance. org**, and the following website allows you to search by state and city, and provides profiles of local Pilates instructors: **http://www. findmypilates.com**.

SELF-TESTS FOR DEPRESSION

There are a variety of tests for depression that can be taken privately to assess your state of depression. It is important, however, to use these self-assessments as tools, not as treatment. The following link discusses a number of available tests and provides several samples:
http://www.depression-help-resource.com/depression-test.htm.

ORGANIZATIONS AND WEBSITES

American Physical Therapy Association
http://www.apta.org

National Association for Continence
http://www.nafc.org

International Continence Society
http://www.continet.org

The Simon Foundation
http://www.simonfoundation.org

Association for Pelvic Organ Prolapse
http://www.pelvicorganprolapsesupport.org

Medline, U.S. National Library of Medicine, National
Institutes of Health
http://www.nlm.nih.gov/medlineplus

National Institutes of Health
http://www.health.nih.gov

National Women's Health Resource Center
http://www.healthywomen.org

National Kidney and Urologic Disease Information
http://www.kidney.niddk.nih.gov

Society for Urodynamics and Female Urology
http://www.sufuorg.com

Insterstitial Cystitis Network
http://www.ic-network.org

The International Pelvic Pain Society
http://www.pelvicpain.org

National Vulvodynia Association
http://www.nva.org

Irritable Bowel Association
http://www.ibsassociation.org

The Whole Woman
http://www.wholewoman.com

WebMD
http://www.webmd.com

American College of Obstetricians and Gynecologists
http://www.acog.org

American Medical Women's Association
http://www.amwa-doc.org

American Urogynecological Society
http://www.augs.org

American Urological Association
http://www.auanet.org

Psychology Resource
http://www.psychology.com

BOOKS

Bologna, R., and Mangano, J. (2006). *The accidental sisterhood: Unlock the power of your secret squeeze*. Pelvic Floor Health, LLC.

Brill, P. (2001). *The core program: 15 minutes a day that can change your life*. New York: Bantam Books.

Gallagher, S., and Kryzanowska, R. (1999). *The Pilates method of body conditioning*. Philadelphia: Bainbridge Books.

Gallagher, S., and Kryzanowska, R. (2000). *The Joseph H. Pilates archive collection*. Philadelphia: Bainbridge Books.

Herrera, I. (2009). *Ending female pain: A woman's manual, the ultimate self-help guide for women suffering from chronic pelvic and sexual pain*. New York: Duplex Publishing.

Hulme, J. (1997). *Beyond Kegels: Fabulous four exercises and more . . . to prevent and treat incontinence*. Missoula, MT: Phoenix Publishing.

Stein, A. (2008). *Heal pelvic pain: A proven stretching, strengthening, and nutrition program for relieving pain, incontinence, IBS, and other symptoms without surgery*. New York: McGraw-Hill.

Wise, D., and Anderson, R. (2006). *A headache in the pelvis: A new understanding and treatment for prostatits and chronic pelvic pain syndromes*. Occidental, CA: National Center for Pelvic Pain Research.

Appendix IV

Shopping List of Discounted Products

The following companies are offering discount pricing for *The Bathroom Key* readers:

■ **StepFree Vaginal Weights**
Set of five weights that build tone and endurance in the pelvic floor, as discussed in Chapter 3.
  Company: SeekWellness
  Phone: 800-840-9301 or 603-574-4921 (Mention *The Bathroom Key* for discount)
  Website: http://www.seekwellness.com/LPs/bathroomkey.htm
  • Use this coupon code when ordering online: **BRKEY0426**

■ **KegelMaster®**
Resistive exercise device (with springs) to increase pelvic floor strength, as discussed in Chapter 3.
  Company: Wellness Partners
  Phone: 888-779-7177 or 916-987-4858 (Mention *The Bathroom Key* for discount)
  Website: http://store.wellnesspartners.com
  • Use this coupon code when ordering online:
    BathroomKeyDis

■ **UTISlip D-Mannose**
A simple sugar that combats urinary tract infections better than cranberry juice, as discussed in Chapter 5.
  Company: Wellness Partners
  Phone: 888-779-7177 or 916-987-4858 (Mention *The Bathroom Key* for discount)

Website: http://store.wellnesspartners.com
- Use this coupon code when ordering online:
  BathroomKeyDis

■ **Magic Circle**

Small piece of resistive Pilates equipment, with accompanying instructional DVD, as discussed in Chapter 6.

Company: Stamina Products, Inc.
Phone: 800-375-7520 (Mention *The Bathroom Key* for discount)
Email: customerservice@staminaproducts.com
- Use this website for discount ordering online:
  http://www.staminaproducts.com/thebathroomkey

■ **AeroPilates Reformers**

For home use with DVD, as discussed in Chapter 6.

Company: Stamina Products, Inc.
Phone: 800-375-7520 (Mention *The Bathroom Key* for discount)
Email: customerservice@staminaproducts.com
- Use this website for discount ordering online:
  http://www.staminaproducts.com/thebathroomkey

■ **Backnobber II® and Jacknobber®**

Tools for self-massage and pressure point relief, as discussed in Chapter 8.

Company: The Pressure Positive Company
Phone: 800-603-5107 or 610-754-6204 (Mention *The Bathroom Key* for discount)
Website: http://www.pressurepositive.com
- Use this coupon code when ordering online:
  BathroomKeyDis

Glossary

Accessory muscles (for continence)   Comprise the transversus abdominus muscle (deep in the trunk), the adductor muscles of the inner thigh, and the gluteal muscles in the buttocks, which assist the pelvic floor muscles in maintaining continence.

Anal sphincter   Inner and outer rings of muscles surrounding the rectum and anus that help to control the passage of gas and bowel movements, along with portions of the pelvic floor muscles.

Anismus   Condition in which the outer (external) anal sphincter and portions of the pelvic floor muscles do not properly relax during defecation, causing constipation and painfully obstructed defecation.

Anus   Muscular opening that is the outlet for bowel movements, located at the end of the rectum.

Bathroom mapping   Knowing where every bathroom is in a given locale, to the point of planning one's outings accordingly.

Behavioral therapy/methods   A nonsurgical, nonpharmacological, noninvasive treatment for incontinence that relies upon exercise, bladder retraining, surface electromyographic (SEMG) biofeedback, coordination training, functional activities, and dietary changes to attain normal bladder function naturally, usually through physical therapy.

Biofeedback   A technique used by physical therapists that allows individuals to see their pelvic floor muscles working on a computer screen. The aim is to normalize the strength, endurance, tone, coordination, and function of these muscles in order to reverse incontinence or other dysfunction, such as pelvic pain or prolapse.

Bladder   Muscular organ located in the pelvis behind the lower abdominals that stores urine until the individual chooses to empty it. *See* **Detrusor muscle.**

Bladder retraining   Type of behavioral therapy that reeducates the bladder naturally, through urge suppression techniques, scheduled voiding, deep breathing, and mind distraction. Urgency, frequency, nocturia, and urge incontinence can all be corrected with bladder retraining.

Bladder suspension surgery   Involves surgically raising the neck of the bladder to correct severe bladder prolapse and a "falling-out" feeling.

Bradley's Loop III   Reflex that governs urinary control. Relaxation of the pelvic floor muscles causes the bladder muscle (detrusor) to contract and empty. Contraction of the pelvic floor muscles encourages the bladder muscle to relax and hold urine.

Cesarean section (C-section)   Procedure in which surgical incisions are made through the mother's abdominal muscles and uterus to deliver the baby through the belly, instead of vaginally.

Cervix   Lowest part of the uterus that forms the top of the vagina. The cervix opens to allow the baby to leave the uterus during vaginal birth.

Chronic pelvic pain   A pelvic pain condition that persists for longer than three months. Pain may be focused in the pelvic floor with referred pain to, or from, local muscles and organs, making an accurate diagnosis challenging. A multidisciplinary approach that includes physical therapy is usually needed.

Clitoris   Organ of female sexual response that extends internally, alongside the front wall of the vagina.

Colon   Stores bowel movements before defecation and connects to the rectum.

Constipation Condition characterized by hard, dry, and firm bowel movements that are difficult to pass. Bowel movement frequency is fewer than three per week.

Continence State in which all urinations take place into the toilet and no involuntary leakage of urine, gas, or fecal matter takes place. The opposite of incontinence.

Contraindication Reasons why a certain medical treatment or procedure should not be administered because the outcome could prove harmful under the circumstances. For example, high-impact exercise is contraindicated in the last trimester of pregnancy.

Core muscles Deepest muscles of the trunk, spine, and pelvis, supporting the spine and organs. These are static postural muscles that do not produce motion.

Cystocele Bulging or dropping of the bladder into the anterior (front) wall of the vagina. Staged from I (least severe) to IV (most severe). *See* **Pelvic organ prolapse.**

Cystogram An x-ray of the bladder.

Cystoscopy Diagnostic procedure involving the insertion of a lit tube into the urethra to view the urethra, bladder, and prostate gland. Samples of tissue (biopsy) or urine can be taken.

Defecate To have a bowel movement.

Depression Major/clinical depression is a mood disorder in which sad, frustrated, or angry feelings interfere with everyday life for extended periods of time.

Detrusor muscle Smooth muscle of the bladder that gives the feeling of urinary urgency and, upon full contraction, empties the bladder of urine.

Diaphragmatic breathing Uses the diaphragm muscle to draw a deeper breath into the lower lobes of the lungs, causing the belly to bulge outward.

Diarrhea Bowel movements of loose or liquid consistency.

Dilator *See* **Vaginal dilator**.

Dyspareunia Painful (or inability to have) sexual intercourse caused by a variety of medical reasons and usually reported only by women. Restrictions and tightness of the pelvic floor muscles are very often a culprit with this condition.

E. coli Bacteria (full name: *Escherichia coli*) found in the urine of ninety percent of women with urinary tract infections (UTIs). Urine should be sterile. *E. coli* are abundant in the lower intestine (as normal flora), but migration to the urethra causes UTIs. Behavioral and hygienic changes can effectively prevent *E. coli* infection of the bladder.

Episiotomy Surgical incision that cuts into the pelvic floor muscles and skin between the vagina and anus to enlarge the vaginal opening during childbirth. The incision can be midline (toward the rectum) or on an angle (medial–lateral). It is a common cause of sexual pain, incontinence, and causes scar tissue in the pelvic floor muscles.

Estrogen Primary female sex hormone that regulates the menstrual cycles and contributes to breast development at puberty.

Fecal incontinence Undesired leakage of bowel movements, causing accidental soiling of clothing or protective padding.

Frequency of urination Voiding urine more often than every three hours throughout the day, even with good hydration. *See* **Hydration**.

Gas incontinence Unintentional expulsion of gas, usually in social situations.

Golgi tendon organ Sensory receptors located in skeletal muscle tendons at insertion into the bone that monitor the tension in the muscle and send signals to the brain.

Hormonal therapy Administration of hormones or chemical substances to treat hormonal deficiencies, as in menopause or hypothyroidism.

Hormone Specialized chemical substances made in endocrine glands (e.g., the thyroid, ovaries, and testes) that regulate metabolism, growth, reproduction, mood, and hunger.

Hydration The supply and utilization of adequate fluids to meet the requirements of biological tissues. One rule of thumb is to divide one's body weight in half and drink that number in ounces on a daily basis.

Hysterectomy Surgical removal of the uterus.

Incontinence (urinary) Any involuntary leakage of urine—large or small, frequent or infrequent. Moderate and severe cases require protective padding to prevent the soiling of outer clothing.

Interstitial cystitis Also called *painful bladder syndrome*, this condition is characterized by urinary urgency and frequency with painful sensations in the bladder and/or pelvis. Interstitial cystitis can also lead to spasms and painful trigger points in the pelvic floor.

Intra-abdominal pressure Occurs within the abdominal cavity, caused by activities such as coughing, lifting, and defecating. Increased intra-abdominal pressure leads to stress urinary and fecal incontinence.

Irritable bowel syndrome A common disorder that involves abdominal pain, cramping, gas, and bloating that has been present for at least six months.

Ischial tuberosities "Sit bones": The pelvic floor muscles attach to these two bony projections on the bottom of the pelvis (ischium), which are felt when sitting.

Kegel, MD, Arnold Henry 1894–1972. An OB/GYN physician and the founding father of pelvic floor muscle training for incontinence. He invented the first pressure-sensing biofeedback device for the pelvic floor, and his name has become synonymous with his exercise approach, which was presented in the late 1940s. He used biofeedback to ensure correct contraction of the pelvic floor muscles, which also gave motivational feedback as incontinence was eliminated.

Kegel exercise The first exercise approach for the pelvic floor, originated by Arnold Kegel, MD.

Key-in-the-door syndrome   A conditioned response characterized by a sudden, uncontrollable urge to urinate the moment one arrives home.

Kidneys   Two glandular organs that filter out waste products from the blood, making urine that is stored in the bladder.

Labia   Comprise the *labia majora*, which are the outer vaginal lips, and the *labia minora*, which are the inner vaginal lips. They serve a protective function around the vagina and urethra.

Levator ani spasms/levator ani syndrome   Spastic involuntary contractions of the pelvic floor muscles that result in pain with sexual intercourse, defecation, and sitting. Often multiple painful trigger points are found in the pelvic floor musculature.

Menopause   The cessation of menstruation, usually occurring between the ages of middle forties to middle fifties.

Mixed urinary incontinence   Stress and urge urinary incontinence occurring together.

Nocturia   Arising from bed to urinate when previously asleep. It is normal to be able to sleep through the night without getting the urge to urinate.

Nocturnal enuresis   Leakage of urine while asleep.

Pelvic brace   Dual contraction of the pelvic floor and the deep transversus abdominus muscles. Together, these muscles reduce intra-abdominal pressure during physical activities, supporting the bladder and preventing stress urinary incontinence.

Pelvic floor   Collective term referring to the group of muscles forming the urogenital hammock of muscles located on the bottom of the pelvis, sometimes referred to as the *pelvic floor muscles* or *pelvic muscles*.

Pelvic floor muscles   Collective term referring to the group of muscles forming the urogenital hammock of muscles located on the bottom of the pelvis, sometimes referred to as the *pelvic floor* or *pelvic muscles*. Pelvic floor muscles do not produce skeletal movement, but they play an important role in continence, organ support, and sexual satisfaction.

Pelvic floor muscles dysfunction   Abnormal or impaired function of the pelvic floor muscles. Symptoms can include incontinence, pain with penetration, or pelvic organ prolapse.

Pelvic floor muscle hypertonicity   Condition in which overactive pelvic floor muscles are held involuntarily in chronic contraction, shortening, and tightness. This high tone interferes with normal function and causes pain, incontinence, and sexual dysfunction.

Pelvic floor muscle incoordination   Lack of coordinated harmonious muscle function that interferes with the pelvic floor's role in defecation, urination, and continence.

Pelvic floor muscle spasm   Involuntary, usually painful, contraction or clenching of the pelvic floor muscles.

Pelvic floor relaxation or release   A technique that eliminates or reduces tone in the pelvic floor muscles, as it facilitates lengthening. It usually combines stretching with bulging or dropping of the pelvic floor muscles during inhalation.

Pelvic organ prolapse   Condition in which organs lose their ligamentous and pelvic floor muscular support, causing them to drop and bulge into the vaginal space. This occurs when the bladder, urethra, rectum, or uterus prolapse into the vagina and are called, respectively, *cystocele, urethracele, rectocele,* and *uterine prolapse.* Four stages diagnose the severity, with Stage I being the least severe and Stage IV being the most severe.

Pelvic pain   Pain that is focused in the pelvic floor and perineum, with referred pain to, or from, local muscles and organs, making an accurate diagnosis challenging. A multidisciplinary approach that includes physical therapy is usually needed.

Perineal body   Central space between the rectum and the vagina. Most of the pelvic floor muscles are attached here.

Perineal tearing   Tears to the skin and pelvic floor muscles around the vaginal opening, occurring during childbirth. Tears are rated from first to fourth degree. A fourth-degree tear is one in which the full thickness of the pelvic floor is torn into the rectum.

Perineometer   Patented in 1951, this was Dr. Arnold Kegel's invention, used to identify and train the pelvic floor muscles to overcome urinary incontinence in women.

Perineum/perineal muscles   Area of pelvic floor muscle and surrounding skin that is between the vagina (or scrotum) and anus, consisting of superficial and deep muscular layers.

Pessary   A small silicone or plastic medical device that is inserted vaginally to treat pelvic organ prolapse and associated incontinence without surgery. There are a wide variety of shapes and sizes, and they are removed periodically for cleaning purposes.

Physical therapist   An individual licensed by the medical board in the state in which he or she practices the profession of physical therapy. There are numerous specialties, and some physical therapists practice exclusively in women's health, helping women overcome their urinary incontinence, pelvic organ prolapse, and pelvic pain.

Physical therapy   A mainstream health care profession that aims to alleviate pain, restore function, and improve the quality of life. There are many specialties.

Pilates, Joseph   1880–1967. Joseph Pilates founded his *Contrology* exercise approach in the early 1900s that later became known as *Pilates*. His ingenious conditioning method targets the deep core muscles that produce better posture, performance, and organ support—the bladder included. Embraced by dancers, athletes, celebrities, physical therapists, their patients, and the general public, its popularity has grown continuously for a century.

Piriformis syndrome   Condition in which the piriformis muscle, a hip muscle located deep within the buttocks that rotates the leg outward, compresses or pinches the adjacent sciatic nerve, causing pain and numbness in the buttock and leg.

Proctalgia fugax   Severe episodic rectal and sacro-coccygeal (tailbone) pain.

Prolapse   *See* **Pelvic organ prolapse**.

Prostadynia   Synonym for **Chronic pelvic pain**.

Pubic bone   Lowest part of the pelvic bone in the front, under the abdomen.

Pudenda nerve   Nerve that supplies the pelvic floor muscles, causing them to voluntarily contract.

Pudendal neuralgia or pudendal nerve entrapment   Condition in which the pudendal nerve becomes compressed, causing chronic stabbing pain, burning, or numbness into the pelvic floor and hip muscles. Pain is often worse with sitting.

Rapid eye movement (REM) sleep   A normal stage of sleep in which the eyes tend to move randomly. It is estimated that humans need 90 to 120 minutes per night of deep REM sleep, because it responsible for archiving memories. Conditions that interfere with a good night's sleep, such as nocturia, should be treated.

Rectocele   Bulging or dropping of the rectum into the posterior (back) wall of the vagina. Staged from I (least severe) to IV (most severe). *See* **Pelvic organ prolapse**.

Rectum   Last portion of the intestines, connecting the colon to the anus.

Resting baseline of the pelvic floor muscles   Amount of tone present in the pelvic floor muscles at rest, as measured by SEMG biofeedback. At rest, the tone should normally be low, but it may be elevated in women with chronic pelvic pain, due to the increased tension in the pelvic floor. Down-training aims to relax the pelvic floor and lower this hypertonicity.

Sacrum   A triangular-shaped bone connecting the lumbar spine with the tailbone and pelvis.

Surface electromyograph (SEMG) biofeedback   Biofeedback technique that does not involve needles. Electrodes read the electrical activity that is produced by the contracting pelvic floor muscles and display this information graphically on a computer screen (similar to an electrocardiograph tracing). This makes rehabilitation of the pelvic floor muscle more motivational and precise, avoiding errors in technique.

Sphincter   Circular muscles around the urethra and anus, with deep (internal) and superficial (external) sections.

Stop test   Stopping or slowing the flow of urine midstream in order to identify and test the strength of the pelvic floor muscles. It is not recommended that this test be repeated more often than once a month to avoid interference with the natural voiding reflex. *See* **Bradley's Loop III**.

Stress incontinence   Leakage of urine associated with activity such coughing, sneezing, lifting, laughing, jumping, running, or moving from a sitting to standing position.

Tantric sex   A type of sexual encounter typified by slow penetration of the penis into the vagina with no movement in the vagina. The man strives to hold back ejaculation by focusing on other sensations, as he remains still. This type of intercourse is helpful for a woman experiencing dyspareunia (painful intercourse), because it allows her pelvic floor muscles to slowly accommodate, thereby reducing the pain.

Transversus abdominus muscle   A deep core muscle (four layers deeper than the rectus abdominus, which is used in sit-up exercises) that attaches under the breastbone (sternum), to the pubic bone, and under all the ribs. It wraps around the waist and connects to the spine in the lower back, resembling a back brace. It gives support to the back, bladder, other organs and is responsible for tall, erect posture and a flat tummy.

Ultrasound   Procedure in which high-frequency sound waves (sonogram) are used for medical imaging of the bladder and urethra. The volume of urine remaining after urination (*post-void residual volume*) can be assessed with ultrasound. A different form of ultrasound is used in the physical therapy clinic and can be used to reduce pelvic pain.

Urethra   Tube through which urine leaves the bladder and exits the body.

Urethrocele Bulging or dropping of the urethra into the anterior (front) wall of the vagina. Staged from I (least severe) to IV (most severe). *See* **Pelvic organ prolapse**.

Urge incontinence Urine leakage that occurs on the way to the bathroom, when the urge to urinate is so strong and so sudden that the person does not make it to the bathroom in time. This is due to an overactive bladder that is in need of retraining.

Urgency of urination An overactive bladder gives stronger, more urgent signals to urinate than normal bladders do. The threat of having an urge-incontinent accident (when the entire bladder empties) is a constant, life-altering source of worry and stress. Certain beverages, such as alcohol, caffeine, and acidic fruit juices, can provoke increased urgency.

Urge suppression techniques Exercise in which the individual remains still, performing five or six strong pelvic floor contractions, thinking of something other than using the bathroom, and taking two deep breaths. This will make the urge to urinate disappear without emptying the bladder. Urge suppression techniques are used when retraining the bladder to empty less often with scheduled voiding.

Urinalysis Test for infection and disease that is performed with a urine sample.

Urinary incontinence Any involuntary leakage of urine—large or small, frequent or infrequent. Moderate and severe cases require protective padding to prevent the soiling of outer clothing.

Urinary retention Condition in which the bladder does not fully empty because of disruption in its contractibility and its coordination with the pelvic floor. Sometimes self-catheterization is necessary until the bladder–pelvic floor coordination is restored.

Urinary tract infection (UTI) Infection of the bladder or urethra, caused by rectal bacteria (*E. coli*) in ninety percent of cases. Urine should be sterile, and infection causes burning with urination. E. coli are abundant in the lower intestine (as normal flora), but migration to the urethra causes UTIs. Behavioral and hygienic changes can effectively prevent *E. coli* infections of the bladder, along with a maintenance dose of D-Mannose.

Urodynamic testing Collective term referring to the many different testing procedures given to assess how well the bladder and urethra are performing their roles of storing and releasing urine. These tests may include postvoid residual volume (amount of urine left in the bladder after urinating), multichannel cystometry (measures pressures in the bladder and rectum using catheters), electromyography of the bladder neck, and fluoroscopy (a moving video x-ray).

Urogynecologist Physician who treats female bladder, uterine, and pelvic floor disorders.

Urologist Physician specializing in urological disorders of the urinary system for both men and women.

Uterine prolapse Dropping or descent of the uterus into the vagina. Staged from I (least severe) to IV (most severe). *See* **Pelvic organ prolapse**.

Uterus Muscular organ that holds the developing fetus during pregnancy.

Vagina Canal spanning from the cervix to the labia.

Vaginal dilator Medical devices made of smooth hard plastic in progressively larger diameters, designed to stretch the pelvic floor muscles at the vaginal opening and deliver trigger point massage.

Vaginismus Pelvic pain condition in which the pelvic floor muscles tense suddenly and involuntarily, making penetration impossible during medical examinations or sexual relations.

Vestibulitis Inflammation and irritation of the vulva; also called *vestibular vulvodynia*.

Void To urinate.

Voiding diary Form on which one writes down daily food and fluid intake, frequency of urination and leakage, and activities causing incontinence, so bladder habits can be assessed and retrained if abnormal. Also called a "Bladder Diary" or "Bladder Log."

Vulva   External female genitalia.

Vulvar vestibulitis   Inflammation and pain of the vulvar vestibule (area between the labia minora containing the urethral and vaginal openings) that causes painful (or inability to have) sexual relations.

Women's Health   Specialty within physical therapy that focuses on treating incontinence, bladder dysfunction, pelvic pain, organ prolapse, and pre- and postpartum rehabilitation.

References

Introduction

Landefeld, S., Bowers, B., Feld, A. D., Hartmann, K. E., et al. (2008). National Institutes of Health state-of-the-science conference statement: Prevention of fecal and urinary incontinence in adults. *Annals of Internal Medicine* 148:449–58.

Zuckerman, G., and Eder, S. (2011). Fund managers juiced about energy stocks. *The Wall Street Journal*, May 13, p. C3.

Chapter 1

http://www.womenshealth.gov/faq/urinary-incontinence.cfm#f

Heaner, M. (2005). Enduring incontinence in silence. *The New York Times*, October 25. http://www.nytimes.com/2005/10/25/health/25inco.html?pagewanted=print (accessed June 24, 2011).

Landefeld, S., Bowers, B., Feld, A. D., Hartmann, K. E., et al. (2008). National Institutes of Health state-of-the-science conference statement: Prevention of fecal and urinary incontinence in adults. *Annals of Internal Medicine* 148:449–58.

Pikul, C. (2011, August 3). Physical Therapy for Your Lady Parts. http://www.oprah.com/health/Womens-Health-Physical-Therapy-Pelvic-Floor-Rehab.

Rogers, G. (2008). Urinary stress incontinence in women. *New England Journal of Medicine* 358:1029–35.

Schuyler, D. (2008). That sinking feeling: Incontinence and other pelvic floor disorders are surprisingly common—But treatable. *The Los Angeles Times*, August 25. http://articles.latimes.com/2008/aug/25/health/he-pelvic25 (accessed June 24, 2011).

Wanli, Y. (2010). Number of incontinence suffers rises in Beijing. *China Daily*, June 30. http://www.chinadaily.com.cn/metro/2010-06/30/content_10039489.htm (accessed June 24, 2011).

Zuckerman, G., and Eder, S. (2011). Fund managers juiced about energy stocks. *The Wall Street Journal*, May 13, p. C3.

Chapter 2

Kegel, A. (1948a). *Nonsurgical method of increasing the tone of sphincters and their supporting structures.* University of Southern California School of Medicine.

Kegel, A. (1948b). Progressive resistance exercise in the functional restoration of the perineal muscles. *American Journal of Obstetrics & Gynecology* 56:238–48.

Kegel, A. (1951). Physiologic therapy for urinary stress incontinence. *Journal of the American Medical Association* 146:915–7.

Monash University. (2011). Regaining control: a new study sheds light on incontinence. September 5. http://www.monash.edu.au/news/show/regaining-control-new-study-sheds-light-on-incontinence (accessed October 3, 2011)

Chapter 3

Barber, M., Dowsett, S. A., Mullen, K., and Viktrup, L. (2005). The impact of stress urinary incontinence on sexual activity in women. *Cleveland Clinic Journal of Medicine* 72:225–32.

Bo, K., Talseth, T., and Vinsnes, A. (2000). Randomized controlled trial on the effect of pelvic floor muscle training on quality of life and sexual problems in genuine stress incontinent women. *Acta Obstetrica et Gynecologica Scandinavica* 79:598–603.

Fox News. (2008, September 25). *Diaper fashion show hits the catwalk.* http://www.foxnews.com/story/0,2933,427822,00.html (accessed June 24, 2011).

Reuters News Service. (2007, February 15). *P&G seeks buyer for Japan adult diaper brand.* http://www.reuters.com/article/2007/02/15/businesspro-pg-japan-diapers-dc-idUST2251820070215 (accessed June 24, 2011).

Chapter 4

Levkowicz, R., Whitmore, K., and Muller, N. (2011). Overactive bladder and nocturia in middle-age American women: Symptoms and impact are significant. *Urologic Nursing* 31:106–111.

Wright, J., and Lenard, L. (2001). D-Mannose & Bladder Infection. Auburn, Washington: Dragon Art. p. 29.

Chapter 5

Burgio, K., Locher, J., Goode, P. S., Hardin, J. M., et al. (1998). Behavioral vs drug treatment for urge urinary incontinence in older women, a randomized controlled trial. *Journal of the American Medical Association* 280:1995–2000.

Kryger, M., Roth, T., et. al (2000). Principles and Practices of Sleep Medicine. Philadelphia: WB Saunders Company. p. 1.572.

Smith, M., Robinson, L., et. al. (2011). helpguide.org/life/sleeping.htm.

Chapter 6

Ellin, A. (2005-07-21). "Now Let Us All Contemplate Our Own Financial Navels." New York Times.

Gallagher, S., and Kryzanowska, R. (2000). *The Joseph H. Pilates archive collection.* Philadelphia, PA: Bainbridge Books.

Gallagher, Sean, PT, Kryzanowska R, (1999). The Pilates® Method of Body Conditioning. Philadelphia: BainBridgeBooks.

Thomson, B. (2003) Joseph Pilates Biography, EasyVigour Project, http://www.easyvigour.net.nz/pilates/h_biography.htm.

Chapter 7

American Urogynecologic Society. (2008). *Pelvic organ prolapse.* http://www.mypelvichealth.org/WhatarePelvicFloorDisorders/PelvicOrgan Prolapse/tabid/126/Default.aspx (accessed June 24, 2011).

Braekken, H., Majida, M., et al. (2010). Can pelvic floor muscle training reverse pelvic organ prolapse and reduce prolapse symptoms? An assessor-blinded, randomized, controlled trial. *American Journal of Obstetrics & Gynecology* 203:e1–7.

Sze, E., and Hobbs, G. (2009). Relation between vaginal birth and pelvic organ prolapse. *Obstetrical & Gynecological Survey* 64:303–4.

U.S. Food and Drug Administration. (2011). *FDA: Surgical placement of mesh to repair pelvic organ prolapse poses risks.* http://www.fda.gov/NewsEvents/Newsroom/Press/Announcements/ucm262752.htm (accessed September 19, 2011).

Writing Group for the Women's Health Initiative Investigators. (2002). Risks and benefits of estrogen plus progestin in healthy post-menopausal women: Principal results of the Women's Health Initiative Randomized Controlled Trial. *Journal of the American Medical Association* 288:321–33.

Chapter 8

Byrne, R. (2006). *The secret.* Hillsboro, OR: Beyond Words Publishing.

Ghaly, A., and Chien, P. (2000). Chronic pelvic pain: Clinical dilemma or clinician's nightmare. *Sexually Transmitted Infections* 76:419–25.

Grace, V. (2000). Pitfalls of the medical paradigm in chronic pelvic pain. *Baillière's Best Practice & Research: Clinical Obstetrics & Gynaecology* 14:525–39.

Herrera, I. (2009). *Ending female pain: A woman's manual, the ultimate self-help guide for women suffering from chronic pelvic and sexual pain.* New York: Duplex Publishing.

Jamieson, D., and Steege, J. (1996). The prevalence of dysmenorrhea, dyspareunia, pelvic pain, and irritable bowel syndrome in primary care practices. *Obstetrics and Gynecology* 87:55–8.

Lampe, A., Sölder, E., Ennemoser, A., Schubert, C., et al. (2000). Chronic pelvic pain and previous sexual abuse. *Obstetrics and Gynecology* 96:929–88.

Mathias, S., Kupperman, M., Liberman, R. F., Lipschutz, R. C., and Steege, J. F. (1996). Chronic pelvic pain: Prevalence, health-related quality of life, and economic correlates. *Obstetrics and Gynecology* 87:321–7.

Reiter, R. (1990). A profile of women with chronic pelvic pain. *Clinical Obstetrics and Gynecology* 33:130–6.

Stein, A. (2008). *Heal pelvic pain: A proven stretching, strengthening, and nutrition program for relieving pain, incontinence, IBS, and other symptoms without surgery.* New York: McGraw-Hill.

Chapter 9

Barber, M., Dowsett, S. A., Mullen, K., and Viktrup, L. (2005). The impact of stress urinary incontinence on sexual activity in women. *Cleveland Clinic Journal of Medicine* 72:225–32.

Bent, A., Cundiff, G. W., and Swift, S. E. (2007). *Ostergard's urogynecology and pelvic floor dysfunction.* Philadelphia: Lippincott Williams & Wilkins.

Brown, W., and Miller, Y. D. (2001). Too wet to exercise? Leaking urine as a barrier to physical activity in women. *Journal of Science and Medicine in Sport* 4:373–8.

Cousins, N. (1981). *Anatomy of an illness as perceived by the patient: Reflections on healing and regeneration.* New York, NY: Bantam.

Gómez-Pinilla, F. (2008). Brain foods: The effects of nutrients on brain function: Nature Reviews Neuroscience 9, 568–578. Doi:10,1038/nrn2421.

Herrera, I. (2009). *Ending female pain: A woman's manual, the ultimate self-help guide for women suffering from chronic pelvic and sexual pain.* New York: Duplex Publishing.

Karg, K., Burmeister, M., Shedden, K., and Sen, S. (2011). The serotonin transporter promoter variant (5-HTTLPR), stress, and depression meta-analysis revisited: Evidence of genetic moderation. *Archives of General Psychiatry* 68:444–54. doi:10.1001/archgenpsychiatry.2010.189.

Melville, J., Fan, M. Y., Rau, H., Nygaard, I. E., and Katon, W. J. (2009). Major depression and urinary incontinence in women: Temporal associations in an epidemiologic sample. *American Journal of Obstetrics & Gynecology* 201:e1–7.

National Institute of Mental Health. (n.d.). *Co-occurrence of depression with heart disease.* http://www.nimh.nih.gov/depression/co_occur/heart.htm (accessed July 1999).

U.S. Department of Health and Human Services. (2008). *Does depression increase the risk for suicide?* http://answers.hhs.gov/questions/3200 (accessed June 24, 2011).

Vigod, S., and Stewart, D. (2006). Major depression in female urinary incontinence. *Psychosomatics* 47:147–51.

Zorn, B., Montgomery, H., Pieper, K., Gray, M., and Steers, W. D. (1999). Urinary incontinence and depression. *Journal of Urology* 162:82–4.

Index